Separation Anxiety in Adulthood

Stefano Pini • Barbara Milrod
Editors

Separation Anxiety in Adulthood

How to Address it in Clinical Practice

Springer

Editors
Stefano Pini
Dept Clinical and Experimental Medicine
University of Pisa
Pisa, Italy

Barbara Milrod
Psychiatry and Behavioral Sc. (PRIME)
Albert Einstein College of Medicine
New York, NY, USA

ISBN 978-3-031-37445-6 ISBN 978-3-031-37446-3 (eBook)
https://doi.org/10.1007/978-3-031-37446-3

This Springer imprint is published by the registered company Springer Nature Switzerland AG
The registered company address is: Gewerbestrasse 11, 6330 Cham, Switzerland

Paper in this product is recyclable.

"My sole consolation when I went upstairs for the night was that Mamma would come in and kiss me after I was in bed. But this good night lasted for so short a time: she went down again so soon that the moment in which I heard her climb the stairs, and then caught the sound of her garden dress of blue muslin, from which hung little tassels of plaited straw, rustling along the double-doored corridor, was for me a moment of the keenest sorrow. So much did I love that good night that I reached the stage of hoping that it would come as late as possible, so as to prolong the time of respite during which Mamma would not yet have appeared. Sometimes when, after kissing me, she opened the door to go, I longed to call her back, to say to her 'Kiss me just once again,' but I knew that then she would at once look displeased, for the concession which she made to my wretchedness and agitation in coming up to me with this kiss of peace always annoyed my father, who thought such ceremonies absurd, and she would have liked to try to induce me to outgrow the need, the custom of having her there at all, which was

a very different thing from letting the custom grow up of my asking her for an additional kiss when she was already crossing the threshold. And to see her look displeased destroyed all the sense of tranquility she had brought me a moment before, when she bent her loving face down over my bed, and held it out to me like a Host, for an act of Communion in which my lips might drink deeply the sense of her real presence, and with it the power to sleep. But those evenings on which Mamma stayed so short a time in my room were sweet indeed compared to those on which we had guests to dinner, and therefore she did not come at all."

Marcel Proust, Swann's Way

Preface

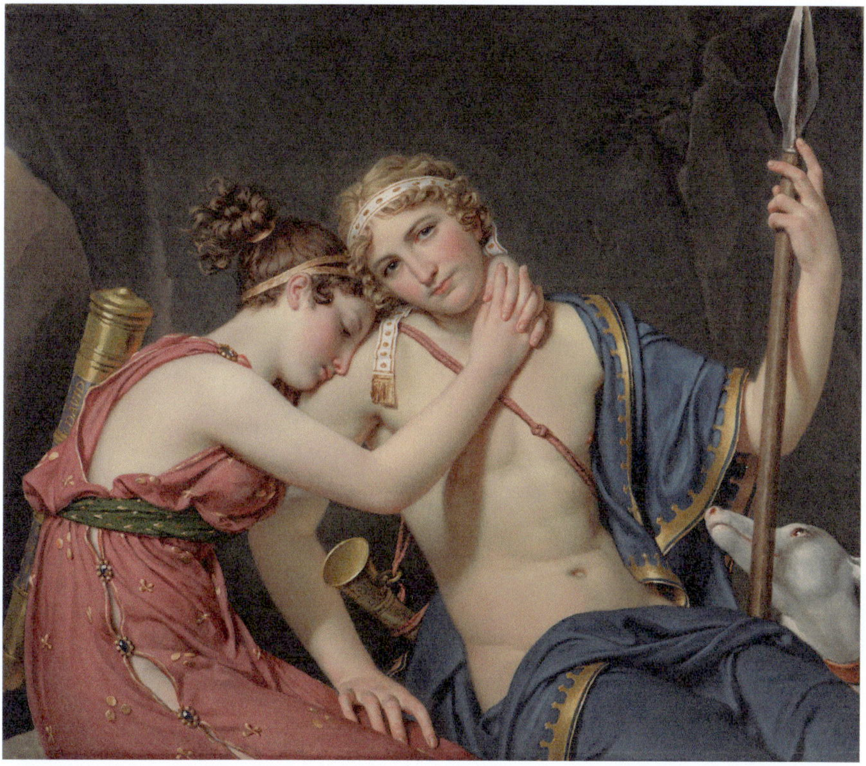

The Farewell of Telemachus and Eucharis, **1818** by Jacques-Louis David. (Digital image courtesy of the Getty's Open Content Program)

The Farewell of Telemachus and Eucharis is a painting from 1818 by Jacques-Louis David, now in the J. Paul Getty Museum in Los Angeles, California. Painted during David's exile in Brussels. The image captures both the sadness and mixed feelings of separation, even in the dog on the right side, gazing at his master and seems to feel and prophesize their separation. Will Telemachus be able to act on his own? Will Eucharis? The painting raises these questions.

Pisa, Italy Stefano Pini
New York, NY, USA Barbara Milrod

Contents

Contributors

Marianna Abelli, MD Department of Clinical and Experimental Medicine, Program of Innovations in Psychiatric Treatments, School of Medicine, University of Pisa, Pisa, Italy

David S. Baldwin, MD Clinical and Experimental Sciences (Clinical Neuroscience), Faculty of Medicine, University of Southampton, Southampton, UK

University Department of Psychiatry and Mental Health, University of Cape Town, Cape Town, South Africa

Mood and Anxiety Disorders Service, Southern Health NHS Foundation Trust, Southampton, UK

Marco Battaglia, MD Centre for Addiction and Mental Health, Toronto, ON, Canada

Department of Psychiatry, University of Toronto, Toronto, ON, Canada

Cundill Centre for Child and Youth Depression, Toronto, ON, Canada

Jill M. Cyranowski, PhD Department of Psychology, University of Pittsburgh, Pittsburgh, PA, USA

John C. Markowitz, MD Columbia University Vagelos College of Physicians and Surgeons, New York, NY, USA

New York State Psychiatric Institute, New York, NY, USA

Vasilios G. Masdrakis, MD Clinical and Experimental Sciences (Clinical Neuroscience), Faculty of Medicine, University of Southampton, Southampton, UK

First Department of Psychiatry, Eginition Hospital, National and Kapodistrian University of Athens Medical School, Athens, Greece

Barbara Milrod, MD Faculty of the New York Psychoanalytic Institute and the Columbia Psychoanalytic Institute for Training and Research, New York, NY, USA

Psychiatry and Behavioral Science (PRIME), Albert Einstein College of Medicine, New York, NY, USA

Laura Molteni, MD Clinical and Experimental Sciences (Clinical Neuroscience), Faculty of Medicine, University of Southampton, Southampton, UK

Luigi Sacco University Hospital, Psychiatry 2 Unit, University of Milan, Milan, Italy

Stefano Pini, MD Department of Clinical and Experimental Medicine, University of Pisa, Pisa, Italy

Accursio Raia, MD Department of Clinical and Experimental Medicine, Program of Innovations in Psychiatric Treatments, School of Medicine, University of Pisa, Pisa, Italy

Gabrielle Silver, MD Weill Cornell Medical College, New York, NY, USA

Maximilian Strauss, MD Centre for Addiction and Mental Health, Toronto, ON, Canada

Introduction to Separation Anxiety: A Guide to the Clinical Syndrome

Barbara Milrod and Stefano Pini

Seemingly newly recognized yet prevalent and ubiquitous, separation anxiety has only been officially acknowledged by the DSM as affecting adults as well as children since the publication of DSM-5 (2013). Yet its prevalence, which varies by country and culture [1] is broad. Its importance has been well-known and well-described for decades [2], particularly if we broaden the strict description of the DSM syndrome a bit to encompass attachment dysregulation and its complicated psychiatric and emotional fallout (see chapter "The Psychodynamic Significance of Separation Anxiety"). Frequently comorbid with other mood and anxiety disorders [1, 3–5], the presence of separation anxiety disorder imparts a worse clinical course, more impairment in role functioning, and decreased efficacy of treatment, regardless of modality, regardless of primary mood or anxiety disorder diagnosis [5–7]. The symptoms of separation anxiety can be overshadowed by other comorbidities, such as mood or other anxiety disorders ([5], see chapter "Clinical Case Descriptions and Discussion" for clinical examples). There is some evidence that improvements in adult separation anxiety [4] and related attachment status [8, 9] may be active mechanisms of change imparted by affect-focused psychotherapies for mood and anxiety disorders, making this a crucial mediator of treatment response to investigate across research domains.

Yet much about the essence and importance of separation anxiety remains murky and inadequately articulated. It is still often ignored clinically. Central questions about the importance of separation anxiety as it affects clinical care of patients

B. Milrod (✉)
Psychiatry and Behavioral Science (PRIME), Albert Einstein College of Medicine, New York, NY, USA
e-mail: bmilrod@montefiore.org

S. Pini
Department of Clinical and Experimental Medicine, University of Pisa, Pisa, Italy
e-mail: stefano.pini@unipi.it

S. Pini, B. Milrod (eds.), *Separation Anxiety in Adulthood*,
https://doi.org/10.1007/978-3-031-37446-3_1

abound: What is the relationship between separation anxiety and attachment status? How much impairment in role functioning and dysregulated relationships engendered by separation anxiety arise from early, more formative central attachment relationship dysregulation, even when separation anxiety is first identified in adulthood [10, 11]? Has the problem of scary, ambivalent attachments been otherwise attributed to "personality disorders" [12], and in what ways will a clearer understanding of separation anxiety alter our clinical approach to these often chronically ill patients who often require care in multiple treatment modalities extending for years, making these patients particularly high utilizers of mental health care? Why does exposure to trauma make separation anxiety worse or does it make separation anxiety present *de novo*? And why has separation anxiety been seemingly systematically ignored within mainstream psychiatry and psychology, except in children, until recently? Most importantly, since the field has ignored this core problem for so long, what are the clinical manifestations of separation anxiety and how can we best address it clinically? Making this task more complicated, there is little large-scale research available to guide either pharmacological or psychotherapeutic interventions for separation anxiety [13].

Panic-Spectrum and Separation Anxiety In 1997, Cassano et al. [14] described pilot testing of the panic-agoraphobic spectrum, a 144-item scale that successfully captures seven domains of symptoms and behavior that characterize patients suffering from panic disorder (PD). High levels of panic-spectrum symptoms, particularly difficulties with separation, contribute to treatment complications and severity of illness, as well as differences between individual patients suffering from PD. One of these core domains is separation anxiety. Worse panic-spectrum symptoms have been shown to be linked to worse therapeutic outcomes in both depression and panic disorder [15]; furthermore, panic-spectrum patients were found to be frequent attenders at medical clinics, resulting in greater medical expenses and more disorganized and attenuated care, often with health anxiety worries that went beyond any medical condition they suffered from [16]. Thus, despite its recent incorporation into our classification systems, separation anxiety seems to contribute to ongoing mental health morbidity and costs.

1 Separation Anxiety Is a Relational Disorder

In contrast to all other mood and anxiety disorders listed in the DSM and ICD, separation anxiety is unique in having symptoms organized in relationship to another individual person or persons. While other anxiety disorders are sometimes characterized by interpersonal difficulties (e.g., social anxiety disorder), separation anxiety disorder is a description of global problems stemming from fears experienced in one or at most a very few individual interpersonal relationships. We describe some of the implications of this problem in greater detail in the chapter "The Psychodynamic Significance of Separation Anxiety", that considers the relationship between separation anxiety and attachment.

It necessarily follows that an essential element of the clinical assessment of separation anxiety must be a clear understanding of how the patient's symptoms affect the other person from whom the patient is anxious when separated from, and their role in the patient's symptoms. Significant clinical differences arise depending on this object's stance on the patient's separation anxiety. Does this other person (as is common in so many cases of childhood separation anxiety, [17]) also experience separation anxiety when apart from the patient, giving rise to and re-enforcing the idea that dangers accrue when they are apart? In mutual self-re-enforcing separation anxiety systems like these, patients may not present for treatment until this mutual anxiety system is threatened, such as what may occur with severe illness or death of the object [18]. Alternatively, is the object of separation anxiety angry at the patient for their controlling, life-limiting anxiety, desperate to break free of the patient's anxiety and the constrictions imposed on their life? (This commonly occurs in teenage children of parents with severe separation anxiety and can lead to counterphobic actions, [17, 19]). Does the other person think the patient's separation anxiety is a problem or do they think it is normal [10]? Ability to engage and success of treatment may depend on these realities about these relationships. Furthermore, the patient's ability to maintain gains acquired in treatment (i.e., greater ability to separate without experiencing crippling anxiety) may depend on changes in the status of this core relationship, and a growing ability for the patient to perceive themselves as safe and able to function without the immediate proximity of the other person.

This book's purpose is to address the questions raised above. Our focus is predominantly clinical, and our goal is to help to guide clinicians to recognize this ubiquitous but understudied psychiatric disorder better, and to articulate approaches to its treatment.

References

1. Silove D, Alonso J, Bromet E, et al. Pediatric-onset and adult-onset separation anxiety disorder across countries in the World Mental Health Survey. Am J Psychiatry. 2015;172:647–56.
2. Baldwin DS, Gordon R, Abelli M, Pini S. The separation of adult separation anxiety disorder. CNS Spectr. 2016;21(4):289–94. https://doi.org/10.1017/S1092852916000080.
3. Elbay RY, Görmez A, Kılıç A, Avcı SH. Separation anxiety disorder among outpatients with major depressive disorder: prevalence and clinical correlates. Compr Psychiatry. 2021;105:152219. https://doi.org/10.1016/j.comppsych.2020.152219. Epub 2020 Dec 19.
4. Milrod B, Keefe JR, Choo TH, Arnon S, Such S, Lowell A, Neria Y, Markowitz JC. Separation anxiety in PTSD: a pilot study of mechanisms in patients undergoing IPT. Depress Anxiety. 2020:1–10. https://doi.org/10.1002/da.23003.
5. Milrod B, Markowitz JC, Gerber AJ, Cyranowski J, Altemus M, Shapiro T, Hofer M, Glatt C. Childhood separation anxiety and the pathogenesis and treatment of adult anxiety. Am J Psychiatr. 2014;171:34–43.
6. Feske U, Frank E, Mallinger AG, Houck PR, Fagiolini A, Shear MK, Grochocinski VJ, Kupfer DJ. Anxiety as a correlate of response to the acute treatment of bipolar I disorder. Am J Psychiatry. 2000;157:956–62.
7. Pini S, Abelli M, Shear KM, Cardini A, Lari L, Gesi C, Muti M, Calugi S, Galderisi S, Troisi A, Bertolino A, Cassano GB. Frequency and clinical correlates of adult separation anxiety

in a sample of 508 outpatients with mood and anxiety disorders. Acta Psychiatr Scand. 2010;122(1):40–6. https://doi.org/10.1111/j.1600-0447.2009.01480.x. Epub 2009 Oct 13.
8. Barber JP, Milrod B, Gallop R, Solomonov N, Rudden MG, McCarthy KS, Chambless DL. Processes of therapeutic change: results from the Cornell-Penn study of psychotherapies for panic disorder. Journal of Counseling Psychology. 2020;67(2):222–31. https://doi.org/10.1037/cou0000417. ISSN: 0022-0167.
9. Markowitz JC, Milrod B, Leuyten P, Holmqvist R. Mentalizing in interpersonal therapy. Am J Psychother. 2019;72:95–100.
10. Milrod B. An epidemiological contribution to clinical understanding of anxiety. Am J Psychiatr. 2015;172:601–2.
11. White LO, Schulz CC, Schoett MJS, Kungl MT, Keil J, Borelli JL, Vrtička P. Conceptual analysis: a social neuroscience approach to interpersonal interaction in the context of disruption and disorganization of attachment (NAMDA). Front Psychiatry. 2020;11:517372. https://doi.org/10.3389/fpsyt.2020.517372. eCollection 2020.
12. Finsaas MC, Klein DN. Adult separation anxiety: personality characteristics of a neglected clinical syndrome. J Abnorm Psychol. 2021;130(6):620–6. https://doi.org/10.1037/abn0000682.
13. Cyranowski J, Milrod B. Separation anxiety disorder in the American Psychiatric Association's textbook of treatments for psychiatric disorders Ed. Gabbard G, editor. Washington, DC: American Psychiatric Press, 2014.
14. Cassano GB, Michelini S, Shear MK, Coli E, Maser JD, Frank E. The panic-agoraphobic spectrum: a descriptive approach to the assessment and treatment of subtle symptoms. Am J Psychiatry. 1997;154(6 Suppl):27–38. https://doi.org/10.1176/ajp.154.6.27.
15. Frank E, Shear MK, Rucci P, Cyranowski JM, Endicott J, Fagiolini A, Grochocinski VJ, Houck P, Kupfer DJ, Maser JD, Cassano GB. Influence of panic-agoraphobic spectrum symptoms on treatment response in patients with recurrent major depression. Am J Psychiatry. 2000;157(7):1101–7. https://doi.org/10.1176/appi.ajp.157.7.1101.
16. Carmassi C, Dell'Oste V, Ceresoli D, Moscardini S, Bianchi E, Landi R, Massimetti G, Nisita C, Dell'Osso L. Frequent attenders in general medical practice in Italy: a preliminary report on clinical variables related to low functioning. Neuropsychiatr Dis Treat. 2019;15:115–25.
17. Preter S, Shapiro T, Milrod B. Child and adolescent anxiety psychodynamic psychotherapy: a manual. Oxford: Oxford University Press; 2018. Print ISBN-13:9780190877712.
18. Milrod B, Shear MK. The psychodynamic treatment of panic disorder. Hosp Community Psychiatry. 1991;42:311–2.
19. Busch F, Milrod B, Singer M, Aronson A. Panic focused psychodynamic psychotherapy: eXtended range: psychodynamic psychotherapy for anxiety disorders: a transdiagnostic treatment manual. Milton Park: Taylor & Francis, LLC; 2012.

Childhood Separation Anxiety: Human and Preclinical Studies

Maximilian Strauss and Marco Battaglia

1 Introduction

Together with the emergence of the separation call, separation anxiety (SA) developed as a defining characteristic of mammalian behaviour [1] and a safety mechanism in newborn mammals, so they would not stray too far from their mothers or safe environments. The convergent evolution of SA in mammals highlights its adaptive function in species survival. However, when behaviour indicates excessive/maladaptive SA, it can be classified as separation anxiety disorder (SAD).

Psychiatry has moved towards recognizing that psychopathological aetiologies do not have one cause, but rather are the result of a complex interplay between genetic predisposition, environmental influences, and cultural characteristics [2–5]. Furthermore, the classification of psychiatric conditions is also subject to cultural, philosophical, and academic influences of the times [4]. The multilayered nature of psychiatric disorders in humans complicates the work of understanding the underlying characteristics and mechanisms for disease. Also, cultural and geographical differences can alter the classification or diagnoses of conditions in different populations, making findings less generalizable [4].

Overall, delineating psychiatric conditions from one another and each of their aetiologies is complicated by clinical classification, and therefore, understanding the mechanistic biology of diseases is desirable for improving the classification and

M. Strauss
Centre for Addiction and Mental Health, Toronto, ON, Canada

M. Battaglia (✉)
Centre for Addiction and Mental Health, Toronto, ON, Canada

Department of Psychiatry, University of Toronto, Toronto, ON, Canada

Cundill Centre for Child and Youth Depression, Toronto, ON, Canada
e-mail: Marco.Battaglia@camh.ca

S. Pini, B. Milrod (eds.), *Separation Anxiety in Adulthood*,
https://doi.org/10.1007/978-3-031-37446-3_2

clinical treatment of mental illnesses. Studying humans is often preferred to understand human disease, particularly psychiatric conditions in which language may play a defining role. However, human studies or clinical trials have inherent practical and ethical limitations embedded into study design and methodology. Using mammalian models as preclinical simulations for understanding psychiatric pathologies can offer solutions to many issues facing investigators and clinicians. Animal models allow investigators to control for factors such as genetics through strain usage, mating, or molecular gene editing. Environmental factors may also be controlled and manipulated in such ways to mimic conditions in which human psychiatric conditions develop. In the context of SAD, mammalian models carry weight due to the common trait of SA in all mammals. Mammalian models also allow for genetic differences be minimized (e.g., via the adoption of inbred strains) amongst subjects exposed to various adversities, and the adversities themselves can be applied with higher consistency. Overall, the use of animal models enables a vast reduction in the variability of experimental conditions, greatly improving generalizability [6].

Another benefit of preclinical animal models is the unique temporal conclusions unattainable in human studies. For example, studying behaviour across generations takes decades in humans, but only months to years in rodents. Using a non-human species with a shorter lifespan, and therefore a shorter timeline for investigation, also poses great benefit to testing the safety and efficacy of therapeutics. Having greater temporal access in such a way allows researchers to better observe the long-term and intergenerational patterns of behaviour and psychopathology.

Animal models, like any model, have limitations. However, the benefits of using animal models repeatedly demonstrate their utility in helping us understand disease in humans, ultimately making up for their shortcomings as a reasonable 'simulation' of a real-world biological system [6, 7].

Needless to say, laboratory animals do not speak, and we know very little of their affective regulation, let alone their individual experiences in a given experimental setting. This means that virtually all behavioural tests of 'anxiety', or 'depression' in preclinical models of human internalizing disorders are inferential. For example, a mouse behaviour on an elevated plus maize (degree of avoidance, time spent in open arms, etc.) is routinely taken as indices of different facets of 'anxiety'. While this is intuitively sensible and empirically legitimate, it is worth remembering that what is really measured in these laboratory settings is a *behaviour*: the next step is the experimenter's interpretation, or labelling, of such behaviour as belonging into 'anxiety', or 'depression'. Since the terms 'anxiety', or 'depression' have a wide terminological halo, semantic short-circuits to human anxiety or depression can easily happen and generate confusion.

Here is where biomarkers, or 'intermediate phenotypes' come to the rescue. Biomarkers in psychiatry are reliable indicators of one or more processes taking place in a specific condition. Biomarker discovery is a crucial avenue in psychiatry meant to improve disease classification, treatment, and future research. An example of the utility of biomarkers in psychiatric progression was in D.F. Klein's pharmacological dissection of 'anxiety neuroses'. Klein showed a differential response of patients with panic disorder (PD) or generalized anxiety disorder (GAD) to tricyclic antidepressants or benzodiazepines, setting up further groups to investigate the similarly split etiology, treatment response, and developmental progression [8–10]. Klein and other groups also showed that PD has developmental continuity with childhood SAD [11–14].

Notably, the biomarker discovery that led to the identification of the SAD-PD continuum indirectly led to the identification of a shared intermediate phenotype of hypersensitivity to carbon dioxide (CO_2) enriched air mixtures [15, 16]. The discovery and understanding of the interconnected SAD, PD, and CO_2 have been investigated by our group. Its development was also made possible through the murine models based on the human clinical findings of SAD-PD relatedness. In this way, the progress we have made has been through a 'human-to-animal and back' framework, a two-way process that can complement the 'bench to bedside' translational framework [17, 18]. The remainder of the chapter will discuss murine mammals' development, validity, applications, and limitations to model SAD, PD, and CO_2 hypersensitivity.

2 SA, SAD, PD, and CO_2 Hypersensitivity in Humans

2.1 Evolutionary Development and Maintenance of Separation Anxiety

The evolutionary development of adaptive separation anxiety is woven throughout mammalian and human evolution. Approximately 4 million years ago marks the first evidence of bipedalism in the genus *Australopithecus* [19]. While walking on two legs suited the environmental pressures of the time, it also required our hominid ancestors to develop a narrower pelvis to enable balance and mobility while engaging in bipedal running [20]. Some 2.5 million years ago, when the *homo* genus separated from that our *Australopithecus africanus* ancestors, the doubling of the human brain and skull size began. Much debate surrounds the cause of the expansion, but regardless of its etiology it is well understood that 2.5 million years ago *homo* brains became larger, we started manufacturing tools, and continued developing more complex brain regions such as the neocortex [21, 22]. The convergence of these properties illustrates a time of cognitive expansion in human history.

With the concurrent expansion of our brains/cognition and the selective pressure pushing for bipedalism, the *homo* genus was subjected to opposing forces driving foetal gestation, maternal birthing, and the child-rearing process [20, 23]. Foetuses had the dual pressure to expand to a larger size throughout childhood and adolescence while also maintaining a 'just right' diameter to ensure the maternal survival of the birthing process [23]. Mothers began birthing increasingly dependent offspring, with foetal cranial diameters and brains that accommodated the constraints of the birth canal and the genus' new neuroanatomy, followed by a period of rapid neural and plastic expansion in childhood [24, 25].

Increasingly premature birthing made *homo* children's better apt at learning complex behaviour, but also more vulnerable, requiring comparatively longer and more complex maternal care for survival [25, 26]. Horses, in contrast, birth foals that can ambulate and explore their environment immediately after delivery. The human neural development and learning period in the following years necessitated a strong mother-infant relationship. Presently, from childhood to adulthood, the volume of the human brain expands by a factor of 3.3, versus a factor of 2.5 in our closest primate ancestors chimpanzees [24]. Uniquely, human brain expansion occurs rapidly in early developmental years rather than consistently throughout a lifetime [25, 27]. While plasticity increased over generations in the children of our ancestors, so did the capacity to explore, practice, and therefore make mistakes necessary to the learning process. Having a strong mother–infant relationship compensated for the consequences of inevitable errors made in the learning processes during childhood [25]. Through the evolutionary balancing act of creating ideal neonate brain volumes, maternal birth canals, and survivability, the stage was set for separation anxiety (SA) to develop as a reciprocal regulator of the mother-infant bond. SA could then mediate a child's return to their mother when exploration and learning became too dangerous [1].

A direct manifestation of SA in newborn mammals is the separation call [28]. In primates, the separation call is a vocalization that maintains mother-offspring contact and is thought to be one of the most ancient forms of mammalian communication. The development of the separation call, alongside nursing and play behaviour, marks the divergence of reptiles from mammals and may have arisen due to the mammalian cingulate and thalamo-cingulate division structures of the brain [1, 29]. In mice, the separation call takes the form of ultrasonic vocalizations (USVs) [28]. In humans, the separation call has corollaries that communicate hunger, pain, and other caregiving urgent demands that are intimately related to survival [1].

2.2 Human SA and SAD

Physiological SA typically enters the repertoire of human behaviour between 6 and 12 months of age and maintains its presence until approximately 3 years of age. Children can form multiple figures of attachment, with the maternal caregiver being the most prominent relationship wherein SA develops [30]. Childhood attachment can extend from the immediate nuclear family to others and is thought to shape separation patterns in adulthood [30].

Childhood SAD is present in approximately 4% of population samples and 7.6% of clinical paediatric samples [31, 32]. It is defined in the Diagnostic and Statistical Manual of Mental Disorders (DSM-V) as the exaggerated or age-inappropriate manifestation(s) of SA [33]. Such categorization implies a degree of continuity between adaptive/useful SA, and the maladaptive/harmful SAD. Childhood SA/SAD are moderately heritable and in a continuum of severity [34]. The causal link between SA and SAD is not definitively understood, but the DSM-V clinically discriminates SA from SAD using eight defining symptoms of SAD [33]. Notably, children may experience a period of heightened or exacerbated SA in response to changing environments that do not necessarily warrant a diagnosis of SAD. Of the eight SAD defining criteria, three symptoms: (1) overt distress related to separation; (2) reluctance to sleep separated from a major attachment figure; and (3) fear of being alone without an attachment figure; best discriminate children with higher versus lower SA [35]. Due to the relationship between SAD and the adult-onset PD and agoraphobia (AGO), it is extremely important to delineate the physiological SA from SAD at a young age. [11, 12]. The median age of onset for SAD is 6, however, it has also been characterized in children as young as 1.5 years old [36, 37].

In an analysis of the Quebec Longitudinal Study of Child Development (QLSCD), we found four distinct trajectories of children with SA [38, 39]. They ranged from a physiological *Low-Persistent* group with minimal SA (60.2% of the sample) to a *High-increasing* group with prominent SA (6.9% of the sample). Of the four trajectories, all but the *high-increasing* group showed a significant symptom reduction by age 4–5. The *high-increasing* group maintained SA from 1.5 to 6 years of age as determined by teacher assessment. The *high-increasing* group was also associated with contextual risk factors such as maternal depression, maternal smoking, and parental unemployment [38]. An early trajectory of high-increasing SA is also associated with multiple negative outcomes later in life. Our follow-up study of the QLCSD children into their mid-childhood and adolescence found the high-increasing SA trajectory associated with: higher internalization, worse academic performance, higher rates of maternal panic/agoraphobia, and higher incidence of adolescent pain, typically headache [40]. The QLSCD data underscore three important themes when discussing SAD: (1) SA and SAD lie on a continuum whereby exacerbated and persistent SA is associated with contextual risk factors and may predict SAD; (2) the use of thresholds on this symptomatic continuum for clinical diagnoses and decision making is necessary to identify children at higher risk of developing SAD and subsequent heterotypic conditions; (3) higher SA appears associated to higher pain/pain sensitivity in adolescence. Regarding the latter two points, the use of clinically observable thresholds, such as teacher- or parental-assessed SA, has its limitations as a clinical determinant of treatment and again highlights the need for a specific and reliable biological or physiological indicator of SAD.

2.3 SAD Continuity with PD and AGO in Humans

A disease spectrum between SAD and PD Agoraphobia (AGO) was first suggested based on clinical observation in the 1990s [11, 15]. Since then the heterotypic continuity between SAD and PD/AGO has long been a topic of debate [41–46]. However, a meta-analysis of 25 studies investigating the link of SAD to other adolescent and adult-onset psychiatric conditions yielded a more definitive statistical link between a childhood diagnosis of SAD to later diagnosis PD/AGO [14]. The analysis used ~15,000 subjects worldwide and demonstrated the specificity of SAD in children predicting PD/AGO later in life with an odds ratio (OR) of 3.45

[2.45–5.0]. The meta-data confirmed earlier findings that SAD, together with a family history of PD/AGO, is a robust predictor of earlier onset PD/AGO, which also indicates an underlying familial-genetic component to the developmental disease spectrum [47, 48]. Notably, no significant relationship was demonstrated between SAD and later depression or substance use. Only other anxiety disorders, pooled, correlated with SAD. However, this was demonstrated by a lower OR of 2.19, highlighting the specificity of SAD to PD-AGO [14].

2.4 Separation Events, Early Life Adversities, and Childhood Parental Loss

SAD patients are described clinically by the DSM-V as experiencing fear of separation [33]. Children with SAD fear and actively avoid benign separation events from attachment figures, often parents. An important topic when discussing SA and SAD is the role of fear of loss vs. actual loss in human SA, SAD, and PD. One form of early life adversity (ELA) is childhood parental loss (CPL). The definition of CPL includes parental death, divorce or separation, or other prolonged separation events such as protracted illness, or military service, before age 17. While the previous CPL separation events are systematized as single-point occurrences, they are more likely to map complex and protracted situations such as, in the instance of parental separation/divorce, conflict and disruption of the family unit that may impact a child's development before the actual loss event occurs. These nuances should be borne in mind when gauging the effects of CPL (or other ELAs) and their contribution to SAD, and when measuring 'real' vs. 'perceived' separation as risk factors.

Independent twin studies have demonstrated CPL as predictor of some (4–5%) phenotypic variance in susceptibility to PD [49, 50]. However, the associations between CPL events and retrospective assessments of childhood SAD have been reported as close to 0 [42, 49]. We have postulated that there may be multiple cascades that CPL may initiate to alter the development of SAD and PD. One cascade (Fig. 1) may occur wherein early CPL predisposes an individual to later develop PD in the absence of clinically defined childhood SAD. An alternative cascade (Fig. 1) could exist such that a child meets the symptomatic criteria for SAD during childhood which later develops into PD [51]. Developmental cascades would be complicated by heritable behavioural traits from parents that create negative childhood rearing environments. Such traits could simultaneously (1) act to disrupt the family's environment preceding a CPL event, and (2) be inherited by the offspring [52].

Regardless of a link between early CPL and SAD in human studies, heritable behavioural factors, such as genetic predisposition to specific behavioural patterns or mental illness, may interact with a child's environment, through CPL or other ELAs, to have a unique synergistic effect on SAD-PD disease progression [53]. This is why it is desirable to identify and quantify the separate effects of gene-environment correlation (rGE) and gene-environment interaction (GxE) to better understand risk processes in childhood SA and develop clinical tools for anxiety disorders [18, 52, 53].

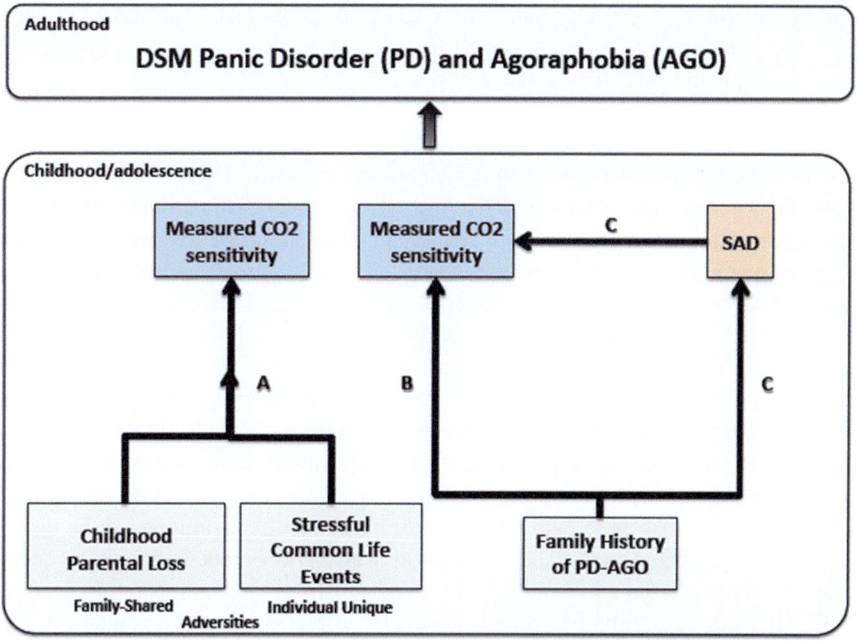

Fig. 1 Differential etiological pathways for developing CO_2 hypersensitivity. **Path A** adversities affect directly CO_2 sensitivity; **Path B** Family History of PD-AGO affects directly CO_2 sensitivity; **Path C**: Family History of PD-AGO affects CO_2 sensitivity via the meditational effect of SAD. PD-AGO, panic disorder-agoraphobia; Family History of PD-AGO: presence of PD-AGO in parents; SAD, Separation Anxiety Disorders by DSM criteria and quantitative measures

2.5 CO_2 Hypersensitivity as an Intermediate Phenotype of SAD and PD/AGO in Humans

While SAD and PD were being recognized as two stages of a shared liability in two different temporal windows, their shared trait of CO_2 hypersensitivity was first described and has been consistently replicated [15, 16, 49, 54–56]. CO_2 constitutes an adverse stimulus across most living organisms, and all mammals—including man—respond to increased CO_2 in inhaled air by enhancing ventilation, arousal, anxiety and by promoting active avoidance of environments high on CO_2 [57].

Human CO_2 hypersensitivity can be operationalised by exaggerated respiratory and/or emotional responses to CO_2-enriched air mixtures that are employed in ad hoc provocation challenges. Several protocols exist that act as a CO_2 respiratory challenge to determine an individual's sensitivity [58]. Of note for distinguishing PD patients from controls, a 35% CO_2–60% O_2 challenge and a 5–7% CO_2 challenge (approximately the physiological concentration in the human lung) have been used. Both protocols have their own characteristics, advantages, and limitations. The 35% CO_2 challenge closely mimics the sudden rise of respiratory symptoms experienced during panic attacks, whereas the 5–7% CO_2 challenge creates a slower onset of anxiety symptoms in sensitive individuals. It has also been shown that the 35% CO_2 challenge may cause a spike in circulating cortisol, suggesting different mechanistic aetiologies for the onset of panic symptoms [59].

The recognition of CO_2 hypersensitivity in both SAD and PD suggests that it can be used as an intermediate phenotype of the two conditions. In the context of SAD and PD, the neurophysiological hypersensitivity to CO_2 in both conditions represents the intermediate phenotype. The utility of an intermediate phenotype arises through investigating its genetic and epigenetic underpinnings, and using those data to explain, model, and treat the two conditions [60]. Our group and others have repeatedly demonstrated the presence of the CO_2 hypersensitivity phenotype in human observational studies of SAD and PD [61, 62]. Additionally, we have shown that genetic traits influence the anxious response to the 35% CO_2 challenge in humans. These effects were distinct from genetic influences of pre-CO_2 baseline anxiety [63]. In twin studies from a Norwegian cohort, we showed that SAD, CO_2 hypersensitivity, and PD co-presentation was 89% influenced by common genetic factors [49, 55].

In the same Norwegian twin cohort, environmental effects influenced the liability of developing SAD and PD. CPL, everyday stressful events, and female gender also reliably predicted a heightened CO_2 hypersensitivity in Campo's twin data set [64]. After correcting the best-fitting model to drop shared environmental effects, except for CPL, we showed that CPL accounted for a significant proportion (11%) of the covariation of SAD, PD and CO_2 hypersensitivity [49]. Consistent with an environmentally influenced etiology for SAD and PD, a meta-analysis of 31,859 twin subjects from the USA, Europe, and Australia found shared environmental and non-shared environmental factors to contribute to 17% and 40% of the difference in SAD presentation, respectively [34].

In a subsequent analysis of gene and environment interaction (a causal interplay whereby environmental factors moderate genetic effects on phenotypic presentation), heightened CO_2 sensitivity was partially explained by a GxE effect, in addition to individual additive effects of genes and non-shared environment, including adversity [53, 65, 66]. Of note, adversity experienced in childhood and adolescence, not during adulthood, explained the GxE effects on CO_2 sensitivity [66].

3 Murine Models of SAD, PD, and CO_2 Hypersensitivity

Mounting evidence that SAD and CO_2 hypersensitivity have shared etiological roots, that SA is present in all mammals, and that responses to CO_2 are amenable to laboratory measurements, make murine SA/SAD modelling particularly valuable. Studying these connections in humans is challenging as the only study design that can be used is naturalistic, which imparts confounds and limitations [17]. Because of the ability to control and manipulate the environment and consistently model adversities, rodent studies can yield an accurate look into the intricacies of the GxE at play in SA/SAD and CO_2 reactivity [6, 7, 17, 65]. The higher population turnover also allows for greater temporal resolution when intergenerational effects are being studied, also enabling study of therapeutic safety and efficacy.

3.1 Murine Modelling of PD Using Early Life Adversities and Neonatal Maternal Separation

Maternal care is crucial to the survival and development of newborn mammals. It follows that suboptimal maternal care, whether its duration truly impacts the care of the newborn pups, acts as a form of early life adversity (ELA). The effect of such ELAs is influenced by the duration and intensity of the adversity, the presence or absence of supportive factors to the newborns, and the developmental stage that the newborn is in. Several protocols exist wherein newborn mice are separated from their mothers with widely varying parameters of separation duration, frequency, and re-uniting [67, 68].

One protocol used to model SA/SAD through maternal separation is the neonatal maternal separation (NMS) method. The protocol operates through separating newborn rat pups from their mothers for 3 h per day consecutively on postnatal days (PND) 3–12. During the daily separation event, the pup is placed in a temperature- and humidity-controlled incubator to prevent any tactile stimulation or interaction with the mother or other pups. Following the 10-day separation protocol, the pup develops under a normal care environment until behavioural and biological measures are taken. The control group for NMS pups are newborns that do not undergo the 3 h separation from PND3-12 [69–71]. The NMS method in rats induces anxiety-like behaviour, causes adults who were separated as pups to exhibit a higher degree of variability in respiratory tidal volume, and a sex-specific change in the respiratory response to enriched CO_2 air mixtures [69, 72, 73]. The sex-specific effect is a 63% greater respiratory response to elevated CO_2 concentration, while males experienced a 47% decrease in respiratory responses when compared to controls. Interestingly, these findings correlate with the higher prevalence of PD in women. Overall, the findings highlight distinct areas of overlap between NMS rats and human PD; namely, parental separation as an ELA and a sex-specific effect on respiratory homeostasis [17].

3.2 NMS Murine Model Mechanisms for Altered Development and CO_2 Response

How NMS exerts its effects on behavioural phenotype is not fully understood. Posited hypotheses include a lack of maternal stimulation, a change in maternal behaviour upon the pups return from separation, and the transmission of stress hormone via maternal milk as underlying factors in neonatal development [74]. In line with a hormonal hypothesis, NMS pups display elevated levels in circulating cortisol 24 h after the last separation period [75]. Circulating cortisol in neonates of this age is typically low, raising the possibility of cortisol-mediated changes in development [74, 76]. NMS also disrupts homeostatic control of the hypothalamus-pituitary-adrenal (HPA) axis by inducing elevated levels of adrenocorticotropic hormone (ACTH) and cortisol. However, these results are sex-specific and only found in female rats. Though a mechanism has not been empirically developed for NMS-mediated developmental changes, it remains possible that cortisol's ability to bind nuclear receptors and alter gene expression during development influence the behavioural phenotype of NMS rats.

Explaining the physiological mechanism relating ELAs with heightened CO_2 sensitivity has grown in interest due to the role that CPL plays in respiratory control, SAD, and PD psychopathology [53, 65, 66, 69, 72, 73]. ELA's negatively affect cognition and behaviour by altering the development of central nervous system (CNS) structures [77–80]. Similarly, NMS rat preparations have shown dysregulated incorporation of baro-, chemo-, and pulmonary receptor afferents as contributing factors to altered CO_2 sensitivity [81, 82]. The differential receptor incorporation occurs by activating the central amygdala in female rats, while in male rats, no CNS-based CO_2 sensitivity change was seen [81–83]. Additionally, these studies demonstrated no change in peripheral chemoreceptor physiology suggesting a central, versus a peripheral, site for NMS pathophysiology [84]. The sex differences in male versus female rats are complicated by sex differences observed in the baroreflex and Hering-Breuer reflexes of anesthetized samples. The differences point towards anesthesia-sensitive neural structures as possible sites for the integration of pathological CO_2 sensitivity [81].

Another site thought to be involved in NMS-mediated CO_2 hypersensitivity is the amygdala [17]. However, this notion is contradicted by data from studies of humans with amygdala lesions. Individuals with bilateral amygdala damage still display panic behaviour in response to the 35% CO_2 challenge [85]. Although it may seem as if the amygdala is not involved, some have interpreted the lesion data to hypothesize that the connectivity between the amygdala and other structures, rather than the amygdala itself, is involved in triggering panic. However, findings in humans and work by other groups also suggest that other CNS structures, such as the medulla oblongata, the brainstem, and the periaqueductal grey matter, are implicated in the CO_2 panic response [10, 61]. Nevertheless, the exact neural mechanism for NMS-mediated CO_2 hypersensitivity has not yet been uncovered and requires further investigation.

3.3 Repeat Cross-Fostering Murine Model of SAD, PD, and CO_2 Hypersensitivity

The NMS protocol is not without limitations. Long-term behavioural and hormonal findings differ between studies, and methodological differences further compound limitations [17, 86, 87]. The repeated cross-fostering (RCF) is another methodology employed to interfere with murine maternal care, that is based on cross-fostering (CF). CF, initially developed for managing pathogen infections in murine lab colonies, entails removing newborn mouse pups from their biological mother and placing them in new cages to be fostered by another lactating female 24–48 h after birth

[88]. Interfering with pup rearing at such an early stage likely interferes with the odour-mediated attachment bonds formed between mother and newborn that signal safety, food, and warmth [89]. Numerous physiological ramifications of CF have been demonstrated and include body weight changes, emotional behaviour differences, metabolic and cardiovascular strain [90–95]. These effects are considered novel changes as they occur while maternal care and nutrition remain sufficient.

The advent of the RCF model, driven by our group, similarly interferes with early maternal bond formation. RCF differs from CF in its repetition of separation events. The methodology takes outbred mouse pups and cross fosters them to new adoptive mothers for 4 days after birth [96]. On PND0 pups (Fig. 2, top) spend the day with their biological mother, then a new adoptive mother every 24 h from PND1 to PND4. During the individual CF events in the PND1-PND4 interval, the mother is initially removed from the cage followed by the litter being removed. The removed litter is then placed into the empty cage of an adoptive mother whose biological pups have recently been removed. The pups are briefly left motherless while the cage is covered in the adoptive mother's bedding. Finally, the adoptive mother is placed in the cage. After the adoptive mother is added to the cage on PND4, there is no change in maternal fostering and normal care routines take place until weaning

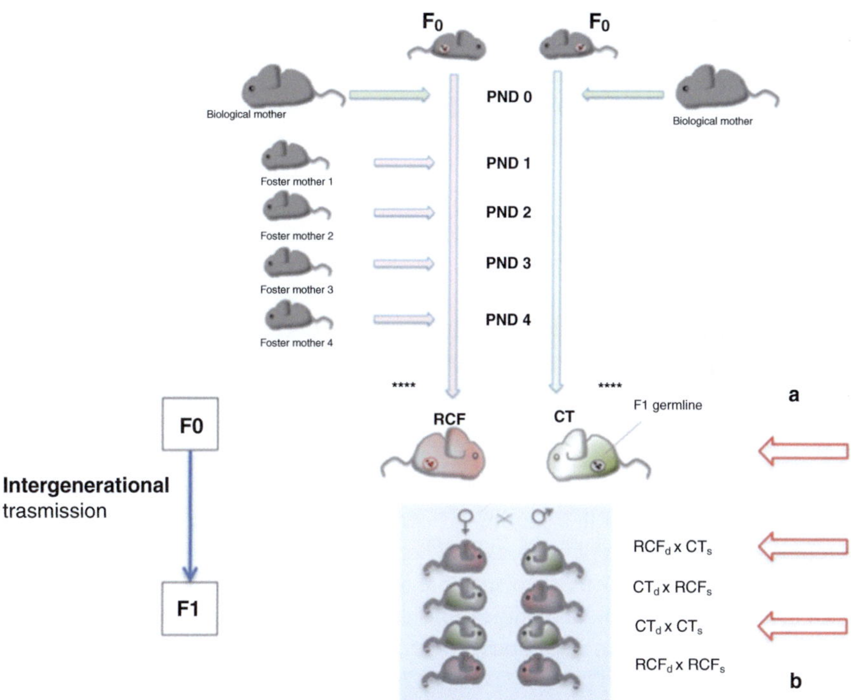

Fig. 2 Graphical description of RCF experimental Design (**a**) RCF procedure (F0 generation); (**b**) Parental crosses to obtain F1 RCF animals. Red arrows depict experimental conditions selected for epigenetic analysis. *PND* Postnatal day, *d* Dams, *s* Sires. (Source: [97])

on PND28. To mitigate differences between RCF pups and controls, control litters are picked up daily, reintroduced into their home cage, semi-covered with home cage bedding, and have their biological mothers returned within 30 s. As well, adoptive mothers are lactating dams who have pups of similar age to their fostered litters [17, 96].

RCF pups on PND8 respond to isolation with heightened ultrasonic calls (the murine equivalent of separation calls) when compared to control pups, a key demonstration of SA-like behaviour. These same pups have an exaggerated hyperventilation response to a 6% CO_2 challenge, which remains from childhood through adulthood, and an avoidance to CO_2 enriched air mixtures [96]. The change in CO_2 response is largely driven by increased tidal volume (a key physiological mechanism to reinstate normal pH in temporarily CO_2-acidified blood). Like humans at the onset of PD [15], RCF pups do not have elevated cortisol levels or altered expression of hippocampal corticosteroid receptors [96, 98]. In contrast, NMS mice display elevated levels of cortisol after the separation protocol [75]. An important finding in RCF pups is the change in genetic variance and heritability of RCF associated increase in tidal volume response to 6%CO_2 stimulation [96]. Increased variance and a nearly two-fold increase in heritability of CO_2 hypersensitivity were found when comparing tidal volume (V_t) during a 6% CO_2 challenge between related cross-fostered (siblings and half-siblings), unrelated cross-fostered, and control mice [96]. The RCF findings are indicative of GxE interactions between RCF as a specific type of ELA and CO_2 hypersensitivity that have been found in human twin studies of CO_2 reactivity [66]. Strengths of the RCF protocol are its non-inferential nature of responses to CO_2 enriched air mixtures and panic-like behaviour [99]. The findings in RCF pups are not limited by unintended procedural consequences either, as maternal care including nursing, licking/grooming behaviour between RCF and control pups does not vary [96]. Later in life, RCF mice display a reduced response to natural rewards and an increased vulnerability to adverse events [100], that may be interpreted as 'depressive-like' behaviour. Overall, from a behavioural and physiological perspective, RCF pups demonstrate reliable CO_2 hypersensitivity and offer insight into the associated illnesses of SA and panic.

3.4 RCF GxE and Epigenetics

The RCF protocol put forth a starting ground to investigate the underlying molecular etiology linking pathophysiology and behaviour linking respiratory physiology, SAD, and PD. Molecular mechanisms that drive GxE and the development of neonates include histone protein modifications and DNA methylation [101]. These epigenetic changes can occur in response to environmental pressures, such as ELAs, to alter gene expression and promote survival of similar challenges in the future [102, 103]. Interestingly, epigenetic signatures do not occur with equal probability across the genome and are correlated with the appearance of new mutations (hence polymorphisms), which potentially carry evolutionary implications [104].

Therefore, it became our goal to understand how environmental ELAs, operationalized in the RCF model, influence epigenetic changes that could be applicable and relevant to human SA, PD and CO_2 sensitivity. In doing so, we would confirm the validity and utility of our model, while simultaneously promoting the treatment of SAD, PD, and other anxiety disorders.

Epigenetic changes were first found through a genome-wide association study (GWAS) of the RCF mouse medulla oblongata, a major site, for the integration of chemoreception and respiratory physiology [105]. The primary histone markers used were H3 acetylation of lysine 9 and 14 (H3Ac), trimethylation of H3 lysine4 (H3K4me3), and trimethylation of lysine 27 (H3K27me3). H3Ac and H3K4me3 indicate gene activation while H3K27me3 indicates gene silencing [106]. The GWAS showed an association of the RCF protocol with enriched histone modification and an extended association with 148 functional enriched genes. Upon transcriptional analysis, enriched genes were identified as belonging to chemoception, nociception, and neurodevelopmental molecular pathways. Of note, the acid-sensing-ion-channel-1 gene *(Asic1)* showed enrichment and increased expression (by both SAGE and rea-time PCR analyses [105]). Acid-sensing ion channels (ASICs), are ubiquitously expressed in the brain (with expression in the medulla oblongata); they mediate pH levels sensing in the blood, as well as nociception, and amygdala-originated fear in response to CO_2 [107, 108].

Consistent with the gene ontology analysis and the theoretical role of ASICs, the RCF mice also showed increased sensitivity to painful stimuli (formalin test), and heightened CO_2 response [105]. A link to human disease can be initially seen through the human ortholog of *asic1* in humans, ACCN2, as it is associated with PD, amygdala function, and CO_2 hypersensitivity [109, 110]. In summary, the RCF model of SA, panic, and CO_2 hypersensitivity demonstrates utility as it: (1) showed that histone modification and ASIC1 are molecular substrates that contribute to a GxE, which may deeply affect the development of SA, nociceptive hypersensitivity, and CO_2 hypersensitivity; (2) set the precedent that future diseases, particularly those that investigate gene-environment interactions, may be effectively understood using controllable murine models and; (3) demonstrated how epigenetic markers may serve in the future as predictors of psychopathology [105].

The epigenetic findings in RCF mice are strengthened from their validation in human study of SA, PD and CO_2 hypersensitivity. When comparing DNA methylation changes from the medulla oblongata of RCF mice to human female monozygotic twin pairs discordant (MZD) for CO_2 hypersensitivity, similar transcriptional regulatory regions and repeated elements were identified [97]. In these investigations RCF mice (F_0) were bred to yield offspring (F_1) who were raised in a normal (no separation or ELAs) environment (Fig. 2, bottom). F_1 mice demonstrated CO_2 hypersensitivity indicating an intergenerational transmission of the RCF induced phenotype [96, 111]. Interestingly, these F_1 medullary changes are consistent with that of RCF(F0) mice and female monozygotic twins who were discordant for CO_2 hypersensitivity. The shared methylation changes were prevalent in genes related to pH acidification homeostasis, chemoreception, anxiety, and neurodevelopment. Amongst these genes, ASIC2 was identified, further strengthening the potential role of ASICs and pH homeostasis in mediating GxE in SA and CO_2 hypersensitivity [97].

The RCF model is useful as it possesses potential as a springboard for therapeutic development and testing. Our group has performed a follow-up study in RCF mice aimed at testing the relevance of ASIC1 in CO_2 responses through pharmacological antagonism [112]. We found that a nebulized dose of ASIC antagonist amiloride, traditionally used to treat high blood pressure, was prophylactically effective in reducing Vt during a 6% CO_2 challenge and thermal pain hypersensitivity [112]. The amiloride data have several implications. First, the success of nebulized amiloride that passes the blood–brain barrier, versus the lack of efficacy of intraperitoneal amiloride, confirms the CNS mediated response to CO_2 enriched air mixtures. Second, the notion that ASICs and acid-sensing play a crucial role in SA and panic was strengthened. Importantly, the validity of RCF as an effective model for human SAD was strengthened.

3.5 Pain, Nociception and Anxiety

It is interesting that McLean's [1] own formulation of the evolutionary relevance of SA included 'pain' amongst the caregiving urgent demands that are conveyed by the separation call, and that our laboratory yielded ASICs-mediated 'altered nociception' amongst the pathways that are most strongly related to the SA-evoking RCF paradigm [97, 105] This calls for a reflection on the relationships between common chronic pain and anxiety in the developmental years.

Chronic pain affects between 8% and 12% of adolescents aged 11–17 years and 16–20% of youth/young adults in North-America and Europe [113, 114]. Adolescent pain is often persistent into adulthood [113–115] and occurs without a recognizable relationship to a medical condition. There is growing epidemiological evidence -echoing similar findings in adults [116] - that childhood/adolescent pain problems are associated with anxiety [40, 117]. While practitioners may be prone to invoke direct causal effects (e.g., pain triggers anxiety, or vice-versa) as a justification (see [118] for a critical appraisal of this simplistic hypothesis), genetic-epidemiological approaches yield alternative, falsifiable explanations. According to our recent systematic review, the majority of twin studies of the co-occurrence of chronic pain and internalizing conditions found substantial covariation of genetic and/or environmental factors as the best-fitting explanation, with only a minority of studies supporting the possibility of phenotypic causation [119]. The only two available twin studies of adolescent pain and anxiety/depression are consistent, and indicate that shared genetic and environmental factors are the most plausible explanation for the co-occurrence of adolescent pain and anxiety/depression [40, 120]. Of relevance, early life adversities including CPL are associated with heightened risk of child/adolescent pain [121] and our preclinical finding of enhanced ASIC-1 expression and altered nociception through epigenetic mechanisms has been independently replicated by preclinical models of perinatal adversities [122].

Pain-anxiety comorbidity also carries important clinical and societal implications. Data suggest that adolescent persistent pain and internalizing disorders may constitute a gateway to premature, more prolonged, and more hazardous opioid prescription [115, 123], in turn a risk for diversion, abuse and possibly overdose [124]. Consistent with these data, the first national US longitudinal analysis of prescription drug misuse indicated that opiate prescriptions in adolescence predict trajectories of substance use and abuse [125]. Taken together, our findings that a single dose of nebulised ASIC antagonist amiloride restores both anxious and nociceptive responses in RCF animals [112] and that amiloride nasal spray shows ideal stability, pharmacokinetic and safety properties [126–128] open some promising potential pharmacological avenues in the treatment of these conditions.

4 Model Limitations and Future Directions

As with all models of biological systems, NMS and RCF models of SAD, PD, and nociceptive hypersensitivity have limitations. In all non-human models, species–species differences exist, as do challenges in assigning human responses to mammalian action, and assessing cognitive, emotional, and behavioural outcomes.

Throughout the development and study of RCF mice, we pursued a mechanistic understanding through which CO_2 hypersensitivity may be linked to adversity and processes underpinning some specific psychiatric conditions [96, 97, 105, 112]. However, the RCF model is limited in that hyperventilation-induced pH changes in the blood alter other behavioural traits and physiological measures, such as blood pressure and heart rate [108]. As well, CO_2 hypersensitivity is neither 100% specific nor comprehensively associated with SAD or PD [10]. Furthermore, some have suggested that differential CO_2 hypersensitivity is indicative of a predisposition to anxiety rather than a novel GxE interaction [129]. Yet multiple analyses suggest otherwise. Genetic factors that influence anxiety pre-CO_2 have been identified and demonstrate independence from other genes enriched by CO_2 challenge [63]. Therefore, it is likely that although there may be some contribution of baseline anxiety to environmentally influenced CO_2 hypersensitivity, the effect cannot be reduced to primarily latent anxiety behaviour. Lastly, individuals with high trait anxiety have demonstrated a proneness to have great subjective responses to placebo conditions [130]. Such responses are not seen in those with heightened reactions CO_2.

In future, the RCF model needs further characterization to better understand the relationships between CO_2 hypersensitivity, SAD, and PD. Specifically, profiling behavioural readouts such as avoidance/preference and exploratory behaviour will yield a more comprehensive understanding of the RCF phenotype [112]. Additionally, the role of ASICs in CO_2 hypersensitivity may be novel but may also be one of multiple mechanisms involved in ELA-enhanced SA. RCF may induce microglial-mediated acid-sensing or inflammatory responses that alter pH homeostasis in the brain, mechanisms which are both being investigated in anxiety disorder (AD) and PD studies [131, 132]. It would be desirable to elucidate the role each mechanism may play in psychiatric respiratory physiology.

Due to the RCF paradigm's induction of altered nociception in addition to CO_2 hypersensitivity, and enhanced SA-like behaviour, another unique avenue of future research lies within understanding the relationship between chronic pain and psychiatric illness [47, 48, 112]. Chronic pain affects over 20% of individuals with mood/anxiety disorders, and its co-presentation in RCF mice carves a potential path for further investigation of these comorbidities, their potentially shared underlying mechanisms, and the role of ASICs and pH-respiratory homeostasis [47, 48, 116]. Lastly, RCF modelling has great implications for human disease. Data generated from amiloride drives the validity of RCF modelling but also serves as a stepping-stone for human pharmacological study [112]. As we demonstrated a dual reduction in CO_2 hypersensitivity and enhanced nociception, a logical next step would be to consider testing nebulized amiloride in human subjects with SAD and PD. Amiloride has been previously used in humans for treatment or experimental treatment of cystic fibrosis and migraine, allowing demonstration of its safety [133, 134]. Furthermore, a recent study suggests that human ASICs have larger effects in cell culture when compared to mouse orthologs, allowing one to theorize that amiloride will not only have an enhanced effect over the RCF mice, but might carry a similar benefit in humans [135].

Finally, we recently demonstrated that the RCF paradigm is associated with enhanced hyperventilation in response to hypercapnia and nociceptive sensitivity among the first generation of RCF-exposed animals, as well as amongst two successive generations of their normally-reared offspring, through matrilineal transmission [136]. This phenotypic transgenerational transmission went hand-in-hand with transgenerational enhancements of ASIC1, ASIC and ASIC3 messenger RNA transcripts in central neurons of the medulla oblongata and the periaqueductal gray matter (two key brain areas for respiration and nociception) of RCF-lineage animals [136]. A single, nebulized dose of amiloride renormalized respiratory and nociceptive responsiveness, again in a transgenerational fashion across the entire RCF lineage [136]. These findings reveal how, following an early-life adversity, a biological memory reducible to a molecular sensor unfolds, shaping adaptation mechanisms over three generations. In addition to being entwined with multiple correlates of human anxiety and pain conditions, our findings indicate nebulized amiloride as a sensible therapeutic avenue.

5 Summary

SA is one of the most ancient mammalian traits, which has the potential to disrupt physiological balance to become pathological and present as SAD. Human studies guided initial insights into the disease, such as its clinical continuity with PD, its external influences from ELAs in childhood, and the respiratory phenotype of heightened CO_2 sensitivity. Studying SAD and PD in humans in this manner can only have limited utility due to inevitable constraints involved in human study. Utilizing mammalian models, such as the NMS and RCF models discussed here, can impart greater clarity and potentially provide new treatment targets. Murine models of SAD/PD play a role in the 'human-to-animal and back' translational framework as they arose from human observational and naturalistic data, develop testing and expansion of study of targets further in mice, for later application and comparison to human disease.

The NMS and RCF models uniquely mimic human disease in their behavioural readouts as well as their presentation of CO_2 hypersensitivity, an intermediate phenotype in human SAD and PD. The current data suggest that CO_2 hypersensitivity is a common trait in both conditions which childhood adversities can influence through a gene-environment interaction mechanism. Furthermore, using an alternate genetic marker identified based on these notions and pharmacological intervention, we have rescued CO_2 hypersensitivity and thermal pain sensitivity induced by RCF. There are many lines of inquiry to follow in the future, but the works presented here suggest that RCF and NMS models may have great utility in the study and potential treatment of human SAD, PD, as well as a potential probe between the link between pain and anxiety disorders. These genetic links can be employed in further guiding human research, biomarker discovery, and therapeutic development and testing.

References

1. MacLean PD. Brain evolution relating to family, play, and the separation call. Arch Gen Psychiatry. 1985;42(4):405–17. https://doi.org/10.1001/archpsyc.1985.01790270095011.
2. Burmeister M, McInnis MG, Zöllner S. Psychiatric genetics: progress amid controversy. Nat Rev Genet. 2008;9(7):527–40. https://doi.org/10.1038/nrg2381.
3. Kendler KS, Zachar P, Craver C. What kinds of things are psychiatric disorders? Psychol Med. 2011;41(6):1143–50. https://doi.org/10.1017/S0033291710001844.
4. Kendler KS. The nature of psychiatric disorders. World Psychiatry. 2016;15(1):5–12. https://doi.org/10.1002/wps.20292.
5. Martin N, Boomsma D, Machin G. A twin-pronged attack on complex traits. Nat Genet. 1997;17(4):387–92. https://doi.org/10.1038/ng1297-387.
6. Ericsson AC, Crim MJ, Franklin CL. A brief history of animal modeling. Mo Med. 2013;110(3):201–5. Retrieved from http://www.ncbi.nlm.nih.gov/pubmed/23829102.
7. Chesselet M-F, Carmichael ST. Animal models of neurological disorders. Neurotherapeutics. 2012;9(2):241–4. https://doi.org/10.1007/s13311-012-0118-9.
8. Hettema JM, Neale MC, Kendler KS. A review and meta-analysis of the genetic epidemiology of anxiety disorders. Am J Psychiatr. 2001;158(10):1568–78. https://doi.org/10.1176/appi.ajp.158.10.1568.
9. Klein DF, Fink MAX. Pychiatric reaction patterns to imipramine. Am J Psychiatr. 1962;119(5):432–8. https://doi.org/10.1176/ajp.119.5.432.
10. Schenberg LC. In: Nardi AE, Freire RCR, editors. A neural systems approach to the study of the respiratory-type panic disorder BT - panic disorder: neurobiological and treatment aspects. Cham: Springer; 2016. https://doi.org/10.1007/978-3-319-12538-1_2.
11. Gittelman Klein R. Is panic disorder associated with childhood separation anxiety disorder? Clin Neuropharmacol. 1995;18. Retrieved from https://journals.lww.com/clinicalneuropharm/Fulltext/1995/18002/Is_Panic_Disorder_Associated_with_Childhood.3.aspx
12. Gittelman R, Klein DF. Relationship between separation anxiety and panic and agoraphobic disorders. Psychopathology. 1984;17(Suppl. 1):56–65. https://doi.org/10.1159/000284078.
13. Klein RG, Koplewicz HS, Kanner A. Imipramine treatment of children with separation anxiety disorder. J Am Acad Child Adolesc Psychiatry. 1992;31(1):21–8. https://doi.org/10.1097/00004583-199201000-00005.

14. Kossowsky J, Pfaltz MC, Schneider S, Taeymans J, Locher C, Gaab J. The separation anxiety hypothesis of panic disorder revisited: a meta-analysis. Am J Psychiatr. 2013;170(7):768–81. https://doi.org/10.1176/appi.ajp.2012.12070893.
15. Klein DF. False suffocation alarms, spontaneous panics, and related conditions: an integrative hypothesis. Arch Gen Psychiatry. 1993;50(4):306–17. https://doi.org/10.1001/archpsyc.1993.01820160076009.
16. Pine DS, Klein RG, Coplan JD, Papp LA, Hoven CW, Martinez J, Kovalenko P, Mandell DJ, Moreau D, Klein DF, Gorman JM. Differential carbon dioxide sensitivity in childhood anxiety disorders and Nonill Comparison Group. Arch Gen Psychiatry. 2000;57(10):960–7. https://doi.org/10.1001/archpsyc.57.10.960.
17. Battaglia M, Ogliari A, D'Amato F, Kinkead R. Early-life risk factors for panic and separation anxiety disorder: insights and outstanding questions arising from human and animal studies of CO_2 sensitivity. Neurosci Biobehav Rev. 2014;46:455–64. https://doi.org/10.1016/j.neubiorev.2014.04.005.
18. Rutter M. Why is the topic of the biological embedding of experiences important for translation? Dev Psychopathol. 2016;28(4pt2):1245–58. https://doi.org/10.1017/S0954579416000821.
19. Leakey MG, Feibel CS, McDougall I, Walker A. New four-million-year-old hominid species from Kanapoi and Allia Bay, Kenya. Nature. 1995;376(6541):565–71. https://doi.org/10.1038/376565a0.
20. Rosenberg K, Trevathan W. Birth, obstetrics and human evolution. BJOG Int J Obstet Gynaecol. 2002;109(11):1199–206. https://doi.org/10.1046/j.1471-0528.2002.00010.x.
21. Rakic P. Evolution of the neocortex: a perspective from developmental biology. Nat Rev Neurosci. 2009;10(10):724–35. https://doi.org/10.1038/nrn2719.
22. Schick KD. Making silent stones speak: human evolution and the dawn of technology/Making Silent Stones Speak. London: Phoenix; 1993.
23. Ponce de León MS, Golovanova L, Doronichev V, Romanova G, Akazawa T, Kondo O, Ishida H, Zollikofer CPE. Neanderthal brain size at birth provides insights into the evolution of human life history. Proc Natl Acad Sci. 2008;105(37):13764–8. https://doi.org/10.1073/pnas.0803917105.
24. DeSilva J, Lesnik J. Chimpanzee neonatal brain size: implications for brain growth in Homo erectus. J Hum Evol. 2006;51(2):207–12. https://doi.org/10.1016/j.jhevol.2006.05.006.
25. Leigh SR. Brain growth, life history, and cognition in primate and human evolution. Am J Primatol. 2004;62(3):139–64. https://doi.org/10.1002/ajp.20012.
26. Leigh SR. Brain ontogeny and life history in Homo erectus. J Hum Evol. 2006;50(1):104–8. https://doi.org/10.1016/j.jhevol.2005.02.008.
27. Martin RD. Human brain evolution in an ecological context (James Arthur lecture on the evolution of the human brain, no. 52, 1982). New York, NY: American Museum of Natural History; 1983.
28. Newman JD. Neural circuits underlying crying and cry responding in mammals. Behav Brain Res. 2007;182(2):155–65. https://doi.org/10.1016/j.bbr.2007.02.011.
29. Panksepp J, Biven L. The archaeology of mind: neuroevolutionary origins of human emotions (Norton series on interpersonal neurobiology). New York: WW Norton & Company; 2012.
30. Ainsworth MDS, Blehar MC, Waters E, Wall S. Patterns of attachment: a psychological study of the strange situation. In: Patterns of attachment: a psychological study of the strange situation. Oxford: Lawrence Erlbaum; 1978.
31. Copeland WE, Angold A, Shanahan L, Costello EJ. Longitudinal patterns of anxiety from childhood to adulthood: the Great Smoky Mountains Study. J Am Acad Child Adolesc Psychiatry. 2014;53(1):21–33. https://doi.org/10.1016/j.jaac.2013.09.017.
32. Ginsburg GS, Becker EM, Keeton CP, Sakolsky D, Piacentini J, Albano AM, Compton SN, Iyengar S, Sullivan K, Caporino N, Peris T, Birmaher B, Rynn M, March J, Kendall PC. Naturalistic follow-up of youths treated for pediatric anxiety disorders. JAMA Psychiatry. 2014;71(3):310–8. https://doi.org/10.1001/jamapsychiatry.2013.4186.
33. American Psychiatric Association. Diagnostic and statistical manual of mental disorders. Washington, DC: American Psychiatric Association; 2013. https://doi.org/10.1176/appi.books.9780890425596.

34. Scaini S, Ogliari A, Eley TC, Zavos HMS, Battaglia M. Genetic and environmental contributions to separation anxiety: a meta-analytic approach to twin data. Depress Anxiety. 2012;29(9):754–61. https://doi.org/10.1002/da.21941.
35. Cooper-Vince CE, Emmert-Aronson BO, Pincus DB, Comer JS. The diagnostic utility of separation anxiety disorder symptoms: an item response theory analysis. J Abnorm Child Psychol. 2014;42(3):417–28. https://doi.org/10.1007/s10802-013-9788-y.
36. Franz L, Angold A, Copeland W, Costello EJ, Towe-Goodman N, Egger H. Preschool anxiety disorders in pediatric primary care: prevalence and comorbidity. J Am Acad Child Adolesc Psychiatry. 2013;52(12):1294–1303.e1. https://doi.org/10.1016/j.jaac.2013.09.008.
37. Shear K, Jin R, Ruscio AM, Walters EE, Kessler RC. Prevalence and correlates of estimated DSM-IV child and adult separation anxiety disorder in the National Comorbidity Survey Replication. Am J Psychiatry. 2006;163(6):1074–83. https://doi.org/10.1176/ajp.2006.163.6.1074.
38. Battaglia M, Touchette É, Garon-Carrier G, Dionne G, Côté SM, Vitaro F, Tremblay RE, Boivin M. Distinct trajectories of separation anxiety in the preschool years: persistence at school entry and early-life associated factors. J Child Psychol Psychiatry. 2016;57(1):39–46. https://doi.org/10.1111/jcpp.12424.
39. Petitclerc A, Boivin M, Dionne G, Zoccolillo M, Tremblay RE. Disregard for rules: the early development and predictors of a specific dimension of disruptive behavior disorders. J Child Psychol Psychiatry. 2009;50(12):1477–84. https://doi.org/10.1111/j.1469-7610.2009.02118.x.
40. Battaglia M, Garon-Carrier G, Côté SM, Dionne G, Touchette E, Vitaro F, Tremblay RE, Boivin M. Early childhood trajectories of separation anxiety: bearing on mental health, academic achievement, and physical health from mid-childhood to preadolescence. Depress Anxiety. 2017;34(10):918–27. https://doi.org/10.1002/da.22674.
41. Aschenbrand SG, Kendall PC, Webb A, Safford SM, Flannery-Schroeder E. Is childhood separation anxiety disorder a predictor of adult panic disorder and agoraphobia? A seven-year longitudinal study. J Am Acad Child Adolesc Psychiatry. 2003;42(12):1478–85. https://doi.org/10.1097/00004583-200312000-00015.
42. Bandelow B, Alvarez Tichauer G, Späth C, Broocks A, Hajak G, Bleich S, Rüther E. Separation anxiety and actual separation experiences during childhood in patients with panic disorder. Can J Psychiatry. 2001;46(10):948–52. https://doi.org/10.1177/070674370104601007.
43. Brückl TM, Wittchen H-U, Höfler M, Pfister H, Schneider S, Lieb R. Childhood separation anxiety and the risk of subsequent psychopathology: results from a community study. Psychother Psychosom. 2007;76(1):47–56. https://doi.org/10.1159/000096364.
44. Hayward C, Wilson KA, Lagle K, Killen JD, Taylor CB. Parent-reported predictors of adolescent panic attacks. J Am Acad Child Adolesc Psychiatry. 2004;43(5):613–20. https://doi.org/10.1097/00004583-200405000-00015.
45. Lewisohn PM, Holm-Denoma JM, Small JW, Seeley JR, Joiner TE. Separation anxiety disorder in childhood as a risk factor for future mental illness. J Am Acad Child Adolesc Psychiatry. 2008;47(5):548–55. https://doi.org/10.1097/CHI.0b013e31816765e7.
46. Silove D, Manicavasagar V, Curtis J, Blaszczynski A. Is early separation anxiety a risk factor for adult panic disorder?: a critical review. Compr Psychiatry. 1996;37(3):167–79. https://doi.org/10.1016/S0010-440X(96)90033-4.
47. Battaglia M, Bertella S, Politi E, Bernardeschi L, Perna G, Gabriele A, Bellodi L. Age at onset of panic disorder: influence of familial liability to the disease and of childhood separation anxiety disorder. Am J Psychiatr. 1995;152(9):1362–4. https://doi.org/10.1176/ajp.152.9.1362.
48. Battaglia M, Bernardeschi L, Politi E, Bertella S, Bellodi L. Comorbidity of panic and somatization disorder: a genetic-epidemiological approach. Compr Psychiatry. 1995;36(6):411–20. https://doi.org/10.1016/S0010-440X(95)90248-1.
49. Battaglia M, Pesenti-Gritti P, Medland SE, Ogliari A, Tambs K, Spatola CAM. A genetically informed study of the association between childhood separation anxiety, sensitivity to CO2, panic disorder, and the effect of childhood parental loss. Arch Gen Psychiatry. 2009;66(1):64–71. https://doi.org/10.1001/archgenpsychiatry.2008.513.

50. Kendler KS, Neale MC, Kessler RC, Heath AC, Eaves LJ. Childhood parental loss and adult psychopathology in women. A twin study perspective. Arch Gen Psychiatry. 1992;49(2):109–16. https://doi.org/10.1001/archpsyc.1992.01820020029004.
51. Battaglia M. Separation anxiety: at the neurobiological crossroads of adaptation and illness. Dialogues Clin Neurosci. 2015;17(3):277–85. Retrieved from: http://www.ncbi.nlm.nih.gov/pubmed/26487808.
52. Rutter M. Environmentally mediated risks for psychopathology: research strategies and findings. J Am Acad Child Adolesc Psychiatry. 2005;44(1):3–18. https://doi.org/10.1097/01.chi.0000145374.45992.c9.
53. Battaglia M. Gene-environment interaction in panic disorder and posttraumatic stress disorder. Can J Psychiatry. 2013;58(2):69–75. https://doi.org/10.1177/070674371305800202.
54. Battaglia M, Ogliari A, Harris J, Spatola CA, Pesenti-Gritti P, Reichborn-Kjennerud T, Torgersen S, Kringlen E, Tambs K. A genetic study of the acute anxious response to carbon dioxide stimulation in man. J Psychiatr Res. 2007;41(11):906–17. https://doi.org/10.1016/j.jpsychires.2006.12.002. Epub 2007 Jan 24. PMID: 17254605.
55. Battaglia M, Pesenti-Gritti P, Spatola CAM, Ogliari A, Tambs K. A twin study of the common vulnerability between heightened sensitivity to hypercapnia and panic disorder. Am J Med Genet B Neuropsychiatr Genet. 2008;147B(5):586–93. https://doi.org/10.1002/ajmg.b.30647.
56. Coryell W, Pine D, Fyer A, Klein D. Anxiety responses to CO2 inhalation in subjects at high-risk for panic disorder. J Affect Disord. 2006;92(1):63–70. https://doi.org/10.1016/j.jad.2005.12.045.
57. Battaglia M. Sensitivity to carbon dioxide and translational studies of anxiety disorders. Neuroscience. 2017;346:434–6. https://doi.org/10.1016/j.neuroscience.2017.01.053.
58. Rassovsky Y, Kushner MG. Carbon dioxide in the study of panic disorder: issues of definition, methodology, and outcome. J Anxiety Disord. 2003;17(1):1–32. https://doi.org/10.1016/S0887-6185(02)00181-0.
59. van Duinen MA, Schruers KRJ, Jaegers E, Maes M, Griez EJL. Hypothalamic–pituitary–adrenal axis function following a 35% CO2 inhalation in healthy volunteers. Prog Neuro-Psychopharmacol Biol Psychiatry. 2004;28(2):279–83. https://doi.org/10.1016/j.pnpbp.2003.10.005.
60. Gottesman II, Gould TD. The endophenotype concept in psychiatry: etymology and strategic intentions. Am J Psychiatry. 2003;160(4):636–45. https://doi.org/10.1176/appi.ajp.160.4.636.
61. Battaglia M, Bertella S, Ogliari A, Bellodi L, Smeraldi E. Modulation by muscarinic antagonists of the response to carbon dioxide challenge in panic disorder. Arch Gen Psychiatry. 2001;58(2):114–9. https://doi.org/10.1001/archpsyc.58.2.114.
62. Roberson-Nay R, Klein DF, Klein RG, Mannuzza S, Moulton JL, Guardino M, Pine DS. Carbon dioxide hypersensitivity in separation-anxious offspring of parents with panic disorder. Biol Psychiatry. 2010;67(12):1171–7. https://doi.org/10.1016/j.biopsych.2009.12.014.
63. Roberson-Nay R, Moruzzi S, Ogliari A, Pezzica E, Tambs K, Kendler KS, Battaglia M. Evidence for distinct genetic effects associated with response to 35% CO_2. Depress Anxiety. 2013;30(3):259–66. https://doi.org/10.1002/da.22038.
64. Ogliari A, Tambs K, Harris JR, Scaini S, Maffei C, Reichborn-Kjennerud T, Battaglia M. The relationships between adverse events, early antecedents, and carbon dioxide reactivity as an intermediate phenotype of panic disorder. Psychother Psychosom. 2010;79(1):48–55. https://doi.org/10.1159/000259417.
65. Battaglia M. Challenges in the appraisal and application of gene–environment interdependence. Eur J Dev Psychol. 2012;9(4):419–25. https://doi.org/10.1080/17405629.2012.689819
.
66. Spatola CAM, Scaini S, Pesenti-Gritti P, Medland SE, Moruzzi S, Ogliari A, Tambs K, Battaglia M. Gene–environment interactions in panic disorder and CO2 sensitivity: effects of events occurring early in life. Am J Med Genet B Neuropsychiatr Genet. 2011;156(1):79–88. https://doi.org/10.1002/ajmg.b.31144.
67. Tractenberg SG, Levandowski ML, de Azeredo LA, Orso R, Roithmann LG, Hoffmann ES, Brenhouse H, Grassi-Oliveira R. An overview of maternal separation effects on behavioural

outcomes in mice: evidence from a four-stage methodological systematic review. Neurosci Biobehav Rev. 2016;68:489–503. https://doi.org/10.1016/j.neubiorev.2016.06.021.
68. Wang D, Levine JLS, Avila-Quintero V, Bloch M, Kaffman A. Systematic review and meta-analysis: effects of maternal separation on anxiety-like behavior in rodents. Transl Psychiatry. 2020;10(1):174. https://doi.org/10.1038/s41398-020-0856-0.
69. Genest S-E, Gulemetova R, Laforest S, Drolet G, Kinkead R. Neonatal maternal separation and sex-specific plasticity of the hypoxic ventilatory response in awake rat. J Physiol. 2004;554(2):543–57. https://doi.org/10.1113/jphysiol.2003.052894.
70. Kinkead R, Gulemetova R, Bairam A. Neonatal maternal separation enhances phrenic responses to hypoxia and carotid sinus nerve stimulation in the adult anesthetized rat. J Appl Physiol (1985). 2005;99(1):189–96. https://doi.org/10.1152/japplphysiol.00070.2005.
71. Kinkead R, Joseph V, Lajeunesse Y, Bairam A. Neonatal maternal separation enhances dopamine D 2 -receptor and tyrosine hydroxylase mRNA expression levels in carotid body of rats. Can J Physiol Pharmacol. 2005;83(1):76–84. https://doi.org/10.1139/y04-106.
72. Kalinichev M, Easterling KW, Plotsky PM, Holtzman SG. Long-lasting changes in stress-induced corticosterone response and anxiety-like behaviors as a consequence of neonatal maternal separation in Long-Evans rats. Pharmacol Biochem Behav. 2002;73(1):131–40. https://doi.org/10.1016/s0091-3057(02)00781-5.
73. Kinkead R, Montandon G, Bairam A, Lajeunesse Y, Horner R. Neonatal maternal separation disrupts regulation of sleep and breathing in adult male rats. Sleep. 2009;32(12):1611–20. https://doi.org/10.1093/sleep/32.12.1611.
74. Macrì S. Neonatal corticosterone administration in rodents as a tool to investigate the maternal programming of emotional and immune domains. Neurobiol Stress. 2016;6:22–30. https://doi.org/10.1016/j.ynstr.2016.12.001.
75. Gulemetova R, Kinkead R. Neonatal stress increases respiratory instability in rat pups. Respir Physiol Neurobiol. 2011;176(3):103–9. https://doi.org/10.1016/j.resp.2011.01.014.
76. Vázquez DM. Stress and the developing limbic-hypothalamic-pituitary-adrenal axis. Psychoneuroendocrinology. 1998;23(7):663–700. https://doi.org/10.1016/s0306-4530(98)00029-8.
77. Buitelaar JK, Huizink AC, Mulder EJ, de Medina PGR, Visser GHA. Prenatal stress and cognitive development and temperament in infants. Neurobiol Aging. 2003;24 Suppl 1:S53–60.; discussion S67–8. https://doi.org/10.1016/s0197-4580(03)00050-2.
78. Charil A, Laplante DP, Vaillancourt C, King S. Prenatal stress and brain development. Brain Res Rev. 2010;65(1):56–79. https://doi.org/10.1016/j.brainresrev.2010.06.002.
79. Fumagalli F, Molteni R, Racagni G, Riva MA. Stress during development: impact on neuroplasticity and relevance to psychopathology. Prog Neurobiol. 2007;81(4):197–217. https://doi.org/10.1016/j.pneurobio.2007.01.002.
80. Graham YP, Heim C, Goodman SH, Miller AH, Nemeroff CB. The effects of neonatal stress on brain development: implications for psychopathology. Dev Psychopathol. 1999;11(3):545–65. https://doi.org/10.1017/S0954579499002205.
81. Dumont FS, Biancardi V, Kinkead R. Hypercapnic ventilatory response of anesthetized female rats subjected to neonatal maternal separation: insight into the origins of panic attacks? Respir Physiol Neurobiol. 2011;175(2):288–95. https://doi.org/10.1016/j.resp.2010.12.004.
82. Kinkead R, Gulemetova R. Neonatal maternal separation and neuroendocrine programming of the respiratory control system in rats. Biol Psychol. 2010;84(1):26–38. https://doi.org/10.1016/j.biopsycho.2009.09.001.
83. Kinkead R, Tenorio L, Drolet G, Bretzner F, Gargaglioni L. Respiratory manifestations of panic disorder in animals and humans: a unique opportunity to understand how supramedullary structures regulate breathing. Respir Physiol Neurobiol. 2014;204:3–13. https://doi.org/10.1016/j.resp.2014.06.013.
84. Soliz J, Tam R, Kinkead R. Neonatal maternal separation augments carotid body response to hypoxia in adult males but not female rats. Front Physiol. 2016;7:432. Retrieved from https://www.frontiersin.org/article/10.3389/fphys.2016.00432.
85. Feinstein JS, Buzza C, Hurlemann R, Follmer RL, Dahdaleh NS, Coryell WH, Welsh MJ, Tranel D, Wemmie JA. Fear and panic in humans with bilateral amygdala damage. Nat Neurosci. 2013;16(3):270–2. https://doi.org/10.1038/nn.3323.

86. Macrì S, Würbel H. Developmental plasticity of HPA and fear responses in rats: a critical review of the maternal mediation hypothesis. Horm Behav. 2006;50(5):667–80. https://doi.org/10.1016/j.yhbeh.2006.06.015.
87. Millstein RA, Holmes A. Effects of repeated maternal separation on anxiety- and depression-related phenotypes in different mouse strains. Neurosci Biobehav Rev. 2007;31(1):3–17. https://doi.org/10.1016/j.neubiorev.2006.05.003.
88. Buxbaum LU, DeRitis PC, Chu N, Conti PA. Eliminating murine norovirus by cross-fostering. J Am Assoc Lab Anim Sci. 2011;50(4):495–9. Retrieved from http://www.ncbi.nlm.nih.gov/pubmed/21838978
89. Landers MS, Sullivan RM. The development and neurobiology of infant attachment and fear. Dev Neurosci. 2012;34(2–3):101–14. https://doi.org/10.1159/000336732.
90. Bartolomucci A, Gioiosa L, Chirieleison A, Ceresini G, Parmigiani S, Palanza P. Cross fostering in mice: behavioral and physiological carry-over effects in adulthood. Genes Brain Behav. 2004;3(2):115–22. https://doi.org/10.1111/j.1601-183X.2003.00059.x.
91. Dickinson AL, Leach MC, Flecknell PA. Influence of early neonatal experience on nociceptive responses and analgesic effects in rats. Lab Anim. 2009;43(1):11–6. https://doi.org/10.1258/la.2007.007078.
92. Leussis MP, Heinrichs SC. Quality of rearing guides expression of behavioral and neural seizure phenotypes in EL mice. Brain Res. 2009;1260:84–93. https://doi.org/10.1016/j.brainres.2009.01.007.
93. Lu L, Mamiya T, Lu P, Niwa M, Mouri A, Zou L-B, Nagai T, Hiramatsu M, Nabeshima T. The long-lasting effects of cross-fostering on the emotional behavior in ICR mice. Behav Brain Res. 2009;198(1):172–8. https://doi.org/10.1016/j.bbr.2008.10.031.
94. Malkesman O, Lavi-Avnon Y, Maayan R, Weizman A. A cross-fostering study in a genetic animal model of depression: maternal behavior and depression-like symptoms. Pharmacol Biochem Behav. 2008;91(1):1–8. https://doi.org/10.1016/j.pbb.2008.06.004.
95. Matthews PA, Samuelsson A-M, Seed P, Pombo J, Oben JA, Poston L, Taylor PD. Fostering in mice induces cardiovascular and metabolic dysfunction in adulthood. J Physiol. 2011;589(16):3969–81. https://doi.org/10.1113/jphysiol.2011.212324.
96. D'Amato FR, Zanettini C, Lampis V, Coccurello R, Pascucci T, Ventura R, Puglisi-Allegra S, Spatola CA, Pesenti-Gritti P, Oddi D, Moles A, Battaglia M. Unstable maternal environment, separation anxiety, and heightened CO2 sensitivity induced by gene-by-environment interplay. PLoS One. 2011;6(4):e18637. https://doi.org/10.1371/journal.pone.0018637.
97. Giannese F, Luchetti A, Barbiera G, Lampis V, Zanettini C, Knudsen GP, Scaini S, Lazarevic D, Cittaro D, D'Amato FR, Battaglia M. Conserved DNA methylation signatures in early maternal separation and in twins discordant for CO2 sensitivity. Sci Rep. 2018;8(1):2258. https://doi.org/10.1038/s41598-018-20457-3.
98. Luchetti A, Oddi D, Lampis V, Centofante E, Felsani A, Battaglia M, D'Amato FR. Early handling and repeated cross-fostering have opposite effect on mouse emotionality. Front Behav Neurosci. 2015;9:93. https://doi.org/10.3389/fnbeh.2015.00093.
99. Spiacci A, Vilela-Costa HH, Sant'Ana AB, Fernandes GG, Frias AT, da Silva GSF, Antunes-Rodrigues J, Zangrossi H. Panic-like escape response elicited in mice by exposure to CO2, but not hypoxia. Prog Neuro-Psychopharmacol Biol Psychiatry. 2018;81:178–86. https://doi.org/10.1016/j.pnpbp.2017.10.018.
100. Ventura R, Coccurello R, Andolina D, Latagliata EC, Zanettini C, Lampis V, Battaglia M, D'Amato FR, Moles A. Postnatal aversive experience impairs sensitivity to natural rewards and increases susceptibility to negative events in adult life. Cereb Cortex. 2013;23(7):1606–17. https://doi.org/10.1093/cercor/bhs145.
101. Feil R, Fraga MF. Epigenetics and the environment: emerging patterns and implications. Nat Rev Genet. 2012;13(2):97–109. https://doi.org/10.1038/nrg3142.
102. Xie L, Korkmaz KS, Braun K, Bock J. Early life stress-induced histone acetylations correlate with activation of the synaptic plasticity genes Arc and Egr1 in the mouse hippocampus. J Neurochem. 2013;125(3):457–64. https://doi.org/10.1111/jnc.12210.

103. Zhou VW, Goren A, Bernstein BE. Charting histone modifications and the functional organization of mammalian genomes. Nat Rev Genet. 2011;12(1):7–18. https://doi.org/10.1038/nrg2905.
104. Battaglia M. Epigenomic landscapes and their relationship to variation, fitness, and evolution. Neurosci Biobehav Rev. 2020;109:90–1. https://doi.org/10.1016/j.neubiorev.2020.01.002.
105. Cittaro D, Lampis V, Luchetti A, Coccurello R, Guffanti A, Felsani A, Moles A, Stupka E, D'Amato FR, Battaglia M. Histone modifications in a mouse model of early adversities and panic disorder: role for Asic1 and neurodevelopmental genes. Sci Rep. 2016;6:25131. https://doi.org/10.1038/srep25131.
106. Barski A, Cuddapah S, Cui K, Roh T-Y, Schones DE, Wang Z, Wei G, Chepelev I, Zhao K. High-resolution profiling of histone methylations in the human genome. Cell. 2007;129(4):823–37. https://doi.org/10.1016/j.cell.2007.05.009.
107. Wemmie JA, Taugher RJ, Kreple CJ. Acid-sensing ion channels in pain and disease. Nat Rev Neurosci. 2013;14(7):461–71. https://doi.org/10.1038/nrn3529.
108. Ziemann AE, Allen JE, Dahdaleh NS, Drebot II, Coryell MW, Wunsch AM, Lynch CM, Faraci FM, Wemmie JA. The amygdala is a chemosensor that detects carbon dioxide and acidosis to elicit fear behavior. Cell. 2009;139(5):1012–21. https://doi.org/10.1016/j.cell.2009.10.029.
109. Savage JE, McMichael O, Gorlin EI, Beadel JR, Teachman B, Vladimirov VI, Hettema JM, Roberson-Nay R. Validation of candidate anxiety disorder genes using a carbon dioxide challenge task. Biol Psychol. 2015;109:61–6. https://doi.org/10.1016/j.biopsycho.2015.04.006.
110. Smoller JW, Gallagher PJ, Duncan LE, McGrath LM, Haddad SA, Holmes AJ, Cohen BM. The human ortholog of acid-sensing ion channel gene ASIC1a is associated with panic disorder and amygdala structure and function. Biol Psychiatry. 2014;76(11):902–10. https://doi.org/10.1016/j.biopsych.2013.12.018.
111. Luchetti A, Battaglia M, D'Amato FR. Repeated cross-fostering protocol as a mouse model of early environmental instability. Bio-Protocol. 2016;6(4):e1734. https://doi.org/10.21769/BioProtoc.1734.
112. Battaglia M, Rossignol O, Bachand K, D'Amato FR, Koninck YD. Amiloride modulation of carbon dioxide hypersensitivity and thermal nociceptive hypersensitivity induced by interference with early maternal environment. J Psychopharmacol. 2018;33(1):101–8. https://doi.org/10.1177/0269881118784872.
113. Dunn KM, Jordan KP, Mancl L, Drangsholt MT, Le Resche L. Trajectories of pain in adolescents: a prospective cohort study. Pain. 2011;152(1):66–73. https://doi.org/10.1016/j.pain.2010.09.006.
114. King S, Chambers CT, Huguet A, MacNevin RC, McGrath PJ, Parker L, MacDonald AJ. The epidemiology of chronic pain in children and adolescents revisited: a systematic review. Pain. 2011;152(12):2729–38. https://doi.org/10.1016/j.pain.2011.07.016.
115. Battaglia M, Garon-Carrier G, Brendgen M, Feng B, Dionne G, Vitaro F, Tremblay RE, Boivin M. Trajectories of pain and anxiety in a longitudinal cohort of adolescent twins. Depress Anxiety. 2020;37(5):475–84. https://doi.org/10.1002/da.22992.
116. McWilliams LA, Goodwin RD, Cox BJ. Depression and anxiety associated with three pain conditions: results from a nationally representative sample. Pain. 2004;111(1–2):77–83. https://doi.org/10.1016/j.pain.2004.06.002.
117. Noel M, Groenewald CB, Beals-Erickson SE, Gebert JT, Palermo TM. Chronic pain in adolescence and internalizing mental health disorders: a nationally representative study. Pain. 2016;157(6):1333–8. https://doi.org/10.1097/j.pain.0000000000000522.
118. Schechter NL. Functional pain: time for a new name. JAMA Pediatr. 2014;168(8):693–4. https://doi.org/10.1001/jamapediatrics.2014.530.
119. Khan WU, Michelini G, Battaglia M. Twin studies of the covariation of pain with depression and anxiety: a systematic review and re-evaluation of critical needs. Neurosci Biobehav Rev. 2020;111:135–48. https://doi.org/10.1016/j.neubiorev.2020.01.015.
120. Scaini S, Michelini G, De Francesco S, Fagnani C, Medda E, Stazi M, Battaglia M. Adolescent pain, anxiety and depressive problems: a twin study of their co-occurrence and the relationship to substance use. Pain. 2022;163(3):e488–94.

121. You DS, Albu S, Lisenbardt H, Meagher MW. Cumulative childhood adversity as a risk factor for common chronic pain conditions in young adults. Pain Med. 2019;20(3):486–94. https://doi.org/10.1093/pm/pny106.
122. Wang H-J, Xu X, Zhang P-A, Li M, Zhou Y-L, Xu Y-C, Jiang XH, Xu G-Y. Epigenetic upregulation of acid-sensing ion channel 1 contributes to gastric hypersensitivity in adult offspring rats with prenatal maternal stress. Pain. 2020;161(5):989–1004. https://doi.org/10.1097/j.pain.0000000000001785.
123. Battaglia M, Quinn PD, Groenewald CB. Consideration of adolescent pain in responses to the opioid crisis. JAMA Psychiatry. 2021;78(1):5–6. https://doi.org/10.1001/jamapsychiatry.2020.1694.
124. Volkow ND, McLellan AT. Opioid abuse in chronic pain — misconceptions and mitigation strategies. N Engl J Med. 2016;374(13):1253–63. https://doi.org/10.1056/NEJMra1507771.
125. McCabe SE, Veliz PT, Dickinson K, Schepis TS, Schulenberg JE. Trajectories of prescription drug misuse during the transition from late adolescence into adulthood in the USA: a national longitudinal multicohort study. Lancet Psychiatry. 2019;6(10):840–50. https://doi.org/10.1016/S2215-0366(19)30299-8.
126. Azzeh M, Battaglia M, Davies S, Strauss J, Dogra P, Yellepeddi V. Novel intranasal treatment for anxiety disorders using amiloride, an acid-sensing ion channel antagonist: pharmacokinetic modeling and simulation. Int J Clin Pharmacol Ther. 2022;60(6):253–63. https://doi.org/10.5414/CP204217. PMID: 35445658.
127. Yellepeddi VK, Battaglia M, Davies SJC, Alt J, Ashby S, Shipman P, Anderson DJ, Rower JE, Reilly C, Voight M, Mim SR. Pharmacokinetics of intranasal amiloride in healthy volunteers. Clin Transl Sci. 2023. https://doi.org/10.1111/cts.13514. Epub ahead of print. PMID: 36932683.
128. Yellepeddi V, Sayre C, Burrows A, Watt K, Davies S, Strauss J, Battaglia M. Stability of extemporaneously compounded amiloride nasal spray. PLoS One. 2020;15(7):e0232435. https://doi.org/10.1371/journal.pone.0232435.
129. Richey JA, Schmidt NB, Hofmann SG, Timpano KR. Temporal and structural dynamics of anxiety sensitivity in predicting fearful responding to a 35% CO2 challenge. J Anxiety Disord. 2010;24(4):423–32. https://doi.org/10.1016/j.janxdis.2010.02.007.
130. Fluharty ME, Attwood AS, Munafò MR. Anxiety sensitivity and trait anxiety are associated with response to 7.5% carbon dioxide challenge. J Psychopharmacol (Oxford, England). 2016;30(2):182–7. https://doi.org/10.1177/0269881115615105.
131. Tay TL, Savage JC, Hui CW, Bisht K, Tremblay M-È. Microglia across the lifespan: from origin to function in brain development, plasticity and cognition. J Physiol. 2017;595(6):1929–45. https://doi.org/10.1113/JP272134.
132. Vollmer LL, Ghosal S, McGuire JL, Ahlbrand RL, Li K-Y, Santin JM, Ratliff-Rang CA, Patrone LG, Rush J, Lewkowich IP, Herman JP, Putnam RW, Sah R. Microglial acid sensing regulates carbon dioxide-evoked fear. Biol Psychiatry. 2016;80(7):541–51. https://doi.org/10.1016/j.biopsych.2016.04.022.
133. Knowles MR, Church NL, Waltner WE, Yankaskas JR, Gilligan P, King M, Edwards LJ, Helms RW, Boucher RC. A pilot study of aerosolized amiloride for the treatment of lung disease in cystic fibrosis. N Engl J Med. 1990;322(17):1189–94. https://doi.org/10.1056/NEJM199004263221704.
134. Tipton AF, Tarash I, McGuire B, Charles A, Pradhan AA. The effects of acute and preventive migraine therapies in a mouse model of chronic migraine. Cephalalgia. 2016;36(11):1048–56. https://doi.org/10.1177/0333102415623070.
135. Xu Y, Jiang Y-Q, Li C, He M, Rusyniak WG, Annamdevula N, Ochoa J, Leavesley SJ, Xu J, Rich TC, Lin MT, Zha X-M. Human ASIC1a mediates stronger acid-induced responses as compared with mouse ASIC1a. FASEB J. 2018;32(7):3832–43. https://doi.org/10.1096/fj.201701367R.
136. Battaglia M, Rossignol O, Lorenzo L-E, Deguire J, Godin AJ, D'Amato FR, De Koninck Y. Enhanced harm detection following maternal separation: transgenerational transmission and reversibility by inhaled Amiloride. Sci Adv. in press 2023.

The Psychodynamic Significance of Separation Anxiety

Gabrielle Silver and Barbara Milrod

Current understanding of the diagnosis of separation anxiety has evolved to encompass people of all ages and developmental stages who suffer from disproportionate worry and fear when faced with separations from close attachment figures. Historically "separation anxiety" was used to describe normative as well as excessive distress in children when separating from parents from infancy onward. By early childhood, the distress from separation anxiety can interfere with a child's ability to explore his/her environment and can limit which activities a child can engage in including typical and expected activities such as attending school. Recently, it has become clearer that in adulthood a resurgence of childhood fears or a new onset of concerns may arise in the context of circumstances experienced as threatening or associated with normal or pathological threats to mortality that also carry with them the threat of separation: such as acknowledging the aging of parents and concern for their well-being as they become infirm or dependent. Separation distress commonly emerges in relation to romantic partners, or as a parent's children grow, become more autonomous, develop, and individuate. This understanding of separation anxiety as manifesting across the developmental spectrum is reflected in the changes in the DSM-5, where for the first time, it is listed among other anxiety disorders, as opposed to being classified as a childhood disorder. Recent research has also uncovered frequent comorbidity with other anxiety disorders [1] as well as mood disorders [2, 3] and less frequently with impulse control disorders [4]. This helps illustrate the psychobiological and developmental consequences, and neuropsychological associations of separation anxiety.

G. Silver (✉)
Weill Cornell Medical College, New York, NY, USA

B. Milrod
Psychiatry and Behavioral Science (PRIME), Albert Einstein College of Medicine, New York, NY, USA
e-mail: bmilrod@montefiore.org

S. Pini, B. Milrod (eds.), *Separation Anxiety in Adulthood*,
https://doi.org/10.1007/978-3-031-37446-3_3

1 Normal Psychobiological Origins of Infant Attachment and Separation Responses

There is an evolving and complex literature over the past century on both normal and dysregulated early childhood attachment and separation anxiety that we use as background for this chapter although we can only briefly summarize it here (see for example [5, 6]). Severe anxiety arising from separation from primary caregivers and attachment figures in early childhood in both mothers and their small infants carries evolutionary advantages for survival among mammals and is adaptive, promoting survival of young and defenseless members of the species, and furthering social cohesion [7–10]. Infant and parent–infant observational studies conducted in the 1940s and 1950s by Anna Freud at the Hampstead War Nurseries and by Margaret Mahler in New York led to the understanding of the developmental process of mother–infant symbiosis, as well as the separation and individuation process necessary for healthy development. D.W. Winicott said "…there is no such thing as an infant, only mother and infant together [11]," highlighting the profound way in which the normative developmental task of infancy and early childhood and of mothers (primary caregivers) is specifically to first become an attached psychological unit and then to use this stable attachment to establish separate, individuated identities. John Bowlby developed the concept of "a secure base" from which a well attached mother–infant dyad produces an infant who can comfortably explore the environment and begin to establish a healthy sense of him/herself as separate from their loving parent who they trust will continue to be there for them on their return (8). Out of this early work a body of literature emerged aimed at elucidating the necessary components of a "good enough" parent–infant attachment pair in which a secure attachment can be established [12–15]. This includes a primary caretaker who is available, responsible, and protective, but not overly controlling, and an infant who is physically able to be held and soothed and develops responses such as a social smile and language such that the relationship is mutually satisfying. These two actors are both affected by their shared and individual environments. Access to sufficient food, shelter, and safety affect both parent and child. Instability of these basic needs as well as the need for nurture can trigger fear and can interfere with normal attachment. The fear system is activated in the service of normal development in various contexts, such as when an infant is passed from a parent's arms to another's, and that infant resists this separation in line with the likelihood that there is in fact a hierarchy of caretakers who are less familiar to the child, and likely decreasingly committed to the well-being of the child. An example of the power of primary attachment relationships and the way they are central in children's learning how to navigate their environment has been termed "social referencing" and has been studied in various contexts [16–18]. An example of this is when a child comes to a precipice such as at the top of a staircase and stops, looking back at their mother in order to better understand the situation and how to act [16]. In a normally developing trusting mother–infant attachment relationship, the infant takes the mother's cues about what is safe and what is not. The typical loving mother will look back with a look of concern, which naturally furthers the child's temporary paralysis keeping the child safe at the top of the stairs and allows the mother time to rush to her side to pick her up or to verbally guide the child toward safer ground. The distracted, or depressed mother may not look at her child at all, thus providing unclear signals to the child about how to proceed. This child may proceed and hurt herself falling down the stairs, or conversely, become overly cautious avoiding stairs altogether, as she cannot trust that anyone is reliably paying attention and would be there to guide her. An insufficient maternal–infant bond, lacking in trust and negotiation of safety, as well as mutual understanding may prepare the ground for an insecurely attached dyad developing into a pathological degree of separation anxiety.

Healthy infants develop a hierarchy of attachment with their primary caretaker, usually the mother, at the top of the hierarchy somewhere around 7 months of age, and they clearly communicate this preference through crying/complaining when separated from that preferred figure.

Clinical Example

Eli was a healthy 7-month-old infant who was sensitive to stimulation and would cry if put down in the crib, however, if held, he would quickly soothe and settle down for sleep. When sitting in the stroller with the cover on he would complain and cry until the cover was lifted, and he could engage with his parent with an exchange of smiles or frowns. When he reached out and mother reached back to touch his hand he would smile with clear pleasure. However, if mother lifted him out of the stroller and tried to pass him to an extended family member or friend he would cry with great seriousness until he was returned to his mother's arms.

Even in the presence of a healthy and normal sense of basic trust developed between parent and child, and normal separation distress, real or fantasied events in which a child (and parent) experience existential threat can activate the fear system and destabilize the sense of "home base" established with "good enough" parenting. No longer does the child feel that the parent can and will protect them from harm. Simultaneously the parent's sense of omnipotence in protecting their child can become quite shaken. This may lead to symptoms of separation anxiety as one or both over-emphasize the need to be together as a way of undoing this new frightening experience of external trauma (war for example).

Clinical Example Continued

At 36 months old Eli had his first serious allergic reaction. He was treated fairly rapidly at home with an antihistamine and alpha agonist and he recovered, although the source of the allergy was unknown. After he experienced a few more moderate allergic reactions, the family had allergy testing done and were able to avoid his consuming the allergenic foods. At age 4, he had a severe allergic reaction at a family gathering requiring the use of an epipen administered by his mother. That fall, Eli was set to begin kindergarten. Every day during the first week of school, Eli became extremely distressed when getting dressed for school, requiring his mother to come in and help dress him, something that did not happen on weekends. He could barely eat breakfast and cried, clinging to his mother at drop off, delaying his entry into the classroom. After a consultation with a child psychiatrist, mother started writing him decorated notes each morning at breakfast that she would put in his lunch box. Also, mother and Eli developed a "special goodbye" where they would hug and mother would sing "mommy comes back, she always comes back to get you," from a video they played at home. By the second week, Eli was able to head off to school with minimal distress.

The physiological response to real threat may be activated in the absence of external threat when there is some dysfunction in the relationship between mother, child, and the environment. The dysfunction may be due to problems with any of the three key elements of the system: infant, mother, or environment, and the ways in which these key elements interact. The degree of severe dysregulation and anxiety experienced by young children when separated for long periods of time from their mothers/caregivers can be so disorganizing as to thwart normal physical and psychological development, in what Rene Spitz termed "anaclitic depression," a condition in which children become utterly withdrawn and fail to thrive [19, 20]. Traumatic environmental circumstances can affect mothers' ability to attach to and care for their small children, and small children can develop post-traumatic syndromes (PTSD) to the degree to which mothers themselves report emotional impairment [21], including depression and emotional effects of trauma [22]. Thus, mothers' emotional stability and emotional health and external circumstances can exert either a protective or a dysregulating impact on small children's emotional adaptation and development of a secure formative attachment [21, 23], prompting the re-framing of Winicott as "there is no such thing as a mother, only a mother and infant in the context of their circumstances [23]."

Maternal capacity for reflective functioning (RF) has been an important area of research in the last 20 years. This concept is closely related to those of internal working models. Reflective functioning in the context of parenting is the capacity to reference the child's mind in one's own mind. In this way a mother may reflect back to a child how his mood or attitude appears through facial expressions, and words so that they share an emotional experience such as joy or frustration. The child, in seeing their inner world reflected back, can organize internally (come to develop his/her own improved reflective capacity of his/her own mind) more readily. This is considered to be a key mediator—from a clinical perspective—in the development of affect regulation [24]. Recent research is elucidating some of the essential elements of reflective functioning, and the different contributions of various primary relationships such as fathers as well as mothers [25]. Halfon and Bekar [26] showed that there was an association between increased use of "mental state words" in which a parent was able to linguistically reflect back on the inner life of the child, to facilitate scaffolding of affect regulation. These mental state words were divided into five categories: (1) emotions, (2) cognitions, (3) perceptions, (4) physiologic, and (5) action. Reflective functioning that engages these five key areas of internal life and shared relationship building is central to the development of trust and the capacity for knowing one's own mind and that of others. A brief child–parent intervention, mothering from the Inside out (MIO) [27, 28] has been developed to improve maternal attunement and attachment to their young children in high risk populations of addicted mothers and mothers who survived abuse in their own childhood. The treatment appears to work by improvements in maternal RF, and has thus far appeared to improve maternal–infant bonding, decreasing separation anxiety and the cycle of abuse.

Clinical Example

Mary was a 2-year-old twin, whose twin sister, Josephine was born with a serious neurologic anomaly requiring repeated surgeries from birth until age 2, with the expectation that she would likely require three or more further procedures as she grew. Both parents were loving parents who very much wanted these children however, mother had a prolonged recovery from the delivery such that she was unable to nurse both girls, and Mary was sent home before mother and Josephine. Both parents had demanding jobs outside the home, and Jo's medical needs were so demanding that both mother and father were quite anxiously engaged in her care leaving little time for Mary. What time they had was shared with great pleasure and mutual engagement. This allowed for Mary to develop as a happy and resilient infant. Mary grew and developed normally until at age 2 ½ her sister had a sudden neurologic event, sending her and their parents to the hospital, which further limited interaction between Mary and her parents due to parental fatigue and the—common enough—parental concept under difficult circumstances like this that Mary "was healthy and fine so needed little from them." Overnight Mary became an irritable, easily disturbed toddler. After mother and Jo returned home Mary stopped talking in public and sobbed and could not be comforted each morning when mother left for work, she became quite aggressive with her twin and with their new baby sister, and she no longer tolerated being dropped off and left to participate in learning activities with other children in her nursery school. Even the babysitter became frustrated as Mary seemed unable to speak, soothe or play unless both parents and siblings were all at home. Parents were at a complete loss and very frustrated that their "healthy child" was now displaying such "pathologic behavior." Although she did not want to come into the office alone initially and did not speak at all for the first few weeks in therapy, the therapist scaffolded Mary's play with the use of narration of what she was doing in her play, and interpreted Mary's silence as a return to her baby years before she "had words when scary things happened, and your sister and parents disappeared." In therapy, after Mary began to speak, the therapist also learned that Mary felt the need to silence herself because of her anger at her sister who "got all the attention." In the following weeks she was increasingly able to engage in the play therapy with words and actions, and at nursery school she began to speak and participate.

While dysregulating anxiety with separation is normal in very young children, if it persists into later childhood and adulthood, or appears anew, it becomes linked to increasingly disrupted perceptions of self and others and carries with it chronic difficulty in maintaining emotional homeostasis and emotion regulation [10] threatening development of normal object relations [29, 30]. Individuals suffering from separation anxiety feel unable to function without the presence of mother or another close attachment figure, without whom the person feels overwhelmed and terrified [7, 8, 10].

Animal (mammalian) models exist of both normative, and dysregulated formative attachment relationships, that presage lifelong emotional difficulties in both rodents and primates [10]. Young rats bred to have high levels of calling responses (a sign of distress) when separated from their mothers showed profound autonomic changes when separated from their mothers. As adults, they were slow to emerge from protective enclosures and showed a passive, "helpless" response to a swim test used to determine "depressive" and "anxious" responses in rodents [31, 32]. Mother bonnet macaques rejected their infants when they were subjected to environmental stressors during pregnancy, specifically, a variable feeding delivery pattern in a laboratory [33–35] . These environmentally stressed mothers had difficulty forming bonds with their infants, remaining distant and distracted, and their offspring were "timid" and were observed to be evidently anxious throughout life [33]. High levels of maternal stress or anxiety appeared to mediate these changes. Early research with human infants and children showed similar findings that of the many factors considered to be important most significant in the development of separation anxiety, maternal anxiety appears to be central [36].

Clinical Example

Kate was an 18-year-old high school senior who had found herself suddenly cut off from friends and teachers during the COVID-19 pandemic when her school shut down. She was now home with her anxious, overly protective mother and pleasantly disengaged father who were also suddenly cut off from their usual routines and social exchanges outside the house at their places of work. Both parents had worked full time throughout Kate's life and had left after dropping her off at school and returned after dinner and bath when she was little, and after dinner as she grew older. Kate had been raised with the help of babysitters. Kate had found intimacy in relationships with babysitters who changed every few years and then with peers at school, in spite of being quite shy and quiet. She had always suffered low levels of social anxiety, but during the social isolation of the pandemic, she found herself anxious all the time. When schools finally re-opened, she was unable to leave her house and had panic attacks if either of her parents left home. At night she stayed up late worrying that one of her parents might die of COVID-19, or of a sudden heart attack, or that an intruder would enter their home and murder all of them. The family had been fortunate enough not to lose anyone due to COVID-19. Some days her worries about everyone's welfare became so overwhelming that she could neither eat nor attend to her schoolwork. Because of her school refusal and crying fits when pressed to leave the house the family sought treatment for her.

In her therapy Kate was able to explore her feelings of loss regarding peers and influential adults outside her home such as teachers, and also to explore her complex mixed feelings about her loving but generally absent parents and the emotional strangeness she had experienced during the period of the pandemic. She was able to explore her ambivalence about graduating from high school and moving on to college. This set of discussions helped her to improve and participate again in school normally.

2 Adult Attachment Style and Separation Anxiety Disorder

The attachment literature and more recent psychiatric and psychological studies pertaining to separation anxiety in adults and children *per se* have largely existed alongside one another as separate-yet related-domains. It makes sense to articulate their relationship here, as these domains share at core the phenomenon of formative early childhood attachment relationships' profound stabilizing, or destabilizing influences on other subsequent attachment relationships, and the related capacity for self-regulation and hence, of overall sense of personal stability. This may bear a relationship to the observed connection between separation anxiety and mood disorders, as noted in the chapter on mood disorders. Scholarship pertaining to attachment style and attachment dysregulation derives originally from careful, mostly psychoanalytic clinical observations and studies of children [6–9, 11, 19, 20], and studies of infant/mother attachment and separation individuation [37, 38]. Adult attachment styles and dysregulation have formed part of the backdrop of psychoanalytic scholarship over the past century [6–9, 11, 19, 20, 37, 39–41], with insecure attachment styles linked to problems in psychic structure formation [41], and to the development of personality disorders [36, 42, 43].

Attachment style in infants aged 9–18 months is described as falling into four categories, depending on how the child responds to a laboratory separation paradigm, described as the Strange Situation, developed by Ainsworth [12]. These categories are operationalized as: securely attached, insecure-avoidant, insecure-ambivalent, and later an insecure-disorganized pattern was described by Main [44]. Maternal attachment status [45] as measured on the adult attachment interview [46] influences child attachment status as measured in the strange situation, although categories of insecure attachment do not necessarily align. Securely attached mothers tend to have securely attached infants, and insecurely attached mothers are likely to have insecurely attached children.

Separation anxiety disorder presents in children with anxious mothers [47], and separation anxiety and other anxiety disorders, particularly social anxiety disorder, in children can emerge as a developmental progression from a profound form of insecure attachment, called "behavioral inhibition" (BI) in young children, in which young children show extreme reticence, avoidance, and fearfulness in new situations [48, 49]. Children with BI were originally identified as being offspring of mothers with panic disorder. Sixty percent of children with BI do not go on to develop lifelong anxiety disorders, so although BI is a genetic and environmental risk factor for later development of severe childhood and later adult anxiety, merging into lifelong social anxiety, other severe anxiety disorders, and timidity, there are evidently protective environmental/epigenetic factors that can correct for this, including very nurturing parenting in rhesus monkey models [50, 51]. Dysregulated fear (DF) at age 2 has been shown to presage childhood separation anxiety at age 4 [52], and it seems clear that insecure early formative attachment relationships, influenced as they are by genetic/neurobiological underpinnings including a lower threshold for limbic and sympathetic nervous system arousal [53] and anxious parenting patterns, including parental inability to manage childhood fears and anxiety [10] play important roles.

Clinical Example

Sara was a 36-year-old married mother of 2. Both of her parents were refugees from separate war-torn countries who had raised Sara in various countries where they were stationed as members of the United States diplomatic corps. She identified with both parental cultures and histories and although she was raised with English as her first language she was multi-lingual. She first presented with depression and extreme anxiety in the context of the birth of her second child. Sara had developed a profound postpartum depression after the birth of her first child and received brief therapy at that time and subsequently, developed a warm although anxious relationship with that toddler. Between births she had suffered from some anxiety and compulsive cleaning but was able to function. She was now terrified that the depression would return and that something terrible would happen to this new infant. She could barely sleep at night, fearful that the newborn would die in her sleep. At the same time her toddler refused to return to his nursery school program and mother was happy to keep him at home where she could keep a watchful eye on both children. Anxiety permeated the household, with Sara frequently terrified about dangers to her children. This time, her husband encouraged her to seek treatment so that she could better manage herself and care for her two children. I initially diagnosed her with postpartum depression and we met for psychodynamic therapy and her depression fairly quickly began to diminish. However, only through a realization that there was an underlying separation anxiety was she able to work through her own frightening childhood experiences in psychotherapy. She had felt prominently and repeatedly abruptly displaced as a child, and over-protected by her vigilant mother; this recognition helped her anxiety to begin to resolve. Then, she was able to encourage her older son to return to nursery school and to put her infant to sleep in a separate room, finally was she able to believe that her infant could survive the night, which had been fuelled by her underlying terror that she herself had confronted, that she might not survive the night.

Maternal anxiety has repeatedly been shown to be associated with the development of separation anxiety in children, but why and in what specific manner this transpires has not been fully explored. Orgiles et al. evaluated parenting style as a mediating factor in the development of separation anxiety in children. They describe an overprotective parenting style which does not allow for children's autonomous function significantly leading to the development of separation anxiety. Punitive and inhibited parenting wherein parents' displayed hostility and/or a lack of support/interest in the individual child was also associated with the development of separation anxiety, while an assertive parenting style in which warmth and autonomy-promoting parenting appeared to be protective for children [54].

3 Psychoanalytic Approach to Separation Anxiety

Ego-Syntonicity Consistent with psychoanalytic ideas about conscious awareness and the ubiquitous presence of unconscious conflict, "separation anxiety" is rarely the presenting complaint of child or adult patients who carry the diagnosis. Many separation anxious children do not bring themselves into treatment, but rather, are brought in by parents who cannot get their child to participate in age-appropriate activities outside the home, or are referred by schools who threaten families with legal intervention if children continue to refuse to attend school. Separation anxious adults are often brought in by romantic partners who cannot tolerate the limitations imposed by their overly anxious partner. The conscious experience of the younger patient may consist of thinking that the danger is circumstantial and that should the circumstance change, they would be fine, not that they are experiencing excessive anxiety. Nonetheless, as children grow older and more socially aware, the sense that they are unable to participate in age-appropriate, normative activities without feeling ill or uncomfortable gradually leads these children and adults to feel incompetent and underlies low self-esteem.

In younger children who deny their anxiety or limitations, the therapist is presented with the need to first collaborate with the patient to understand the arc of their worries so that together they can first observe conscious worries, and later begin to explore the unconscious underpinnings of those worries. For a 4-year-old child who fears that something terrible will happen to her parent if she is separated from them, being dropped off at nursery school may feel dangerous and impossible. Of course, even this carries with it a sense of disappointment in herself. Similarly, a newly married refugee who suffered great emotional and material losses in reaching his adopted country may feel quite destabilized when his wife flies across the country for a week-long conference. Both of these individuals may feel that the solution is simple: don't go to school, stay home and learn; or discourage your new wife from attending the conference. These solutions may be complied with, the anxiety relieved briefly in the short run, and therefore not experienced as necessarily problematic moving forward by the patient. Only when the parent or other attachment figure refuses to comply with these solutions, or when the demands of separation anxiety become a repeated and enraging burden on attachment figures will the symptoms of anxiety emerge as more symptomatic of a full-blown disorder that requires treatment.

Often the unconscious conflict underlying separation anxiety concerns a wish for normal developmentally progressive independence which comes into conflict with unresolved developmental, or traumatic elements of formative relationships that encourage a (regressive) need to be physically close to important attachment figure(s). A child may be sensitive to mother's excessive anxiety that something bad will happen to her if she leaves mother's sight and therefore repress her own normative desire to explore the world in order to soothe or somehow care for the anxious mother. Another common underlying emotional underpinning to separation anxiety might be a child who has never felt sufficiently loved because his parent is absent, who cannot move to the next normative developmental phase which involves increasing focus on relationships with teachers and peers because he is still—possibly unconsciously—seeking parental attention that is out of reach. The dynamic understanding of the mental processes underlying separation anxiety is affirmed by research that has associated environmental factors such as parental loss, extended parental absences, severe parental anxiety, parental alcoholism, low parental warmth and parenting styles that discourage the development of autonomy with the development of separation anxiety [6, 22, 23, 36, 55, 56]. Adult separation anxiety appears to emerge apparently de novo, when it does, or as a recrudescence of earlier struggles with insecure attachment, during times of either new or revived insecure attachment, such as after severe illness or overwhelming trauma, or at times reminiscent of earlier formative attachment insecurities [2, 3, 57].

Psychoanalysts in approaching such patients seek to understand genetic (i.e., developmentally historical) sources of current experiences. Children internalize early experiences and respond in ways that may have been adaptive in early circumstances, but may be maladaptive later in life [10]. For example, if an infant learns that a distracted parent will come if he screams and cries, he may learn to scream and cry when he is lonely or anxious. Attachment behaviors that promote proximity between infant and caretaker or adult and beloved other may be maladaptive in the context of healthy demands for independence and autonomy. For example, it would ultimately feel more empowering for a child and parent if the child could develop healthier means of getting a parent's attention such as putting on a show or playing catch rather than throwing a tantrum. The presence of these behaviors in inappropriate circumstances constitute "symptoms." These symptoms, such as clinging, or refusing to leave the house, may feel safer than acknowledging conflicting wishes for greater independence and unmet needs for love and security [58].

Separation anxious patients may defend against feelings such as anger or disappointment with a parent who cannot sufficiently soothe them by worrying that something bad will happen to that parent, thereby protecting themselves from the painful or difficult awareness of their anger and substituting it with worry for the parent's safety. Another patient may defend against the feeling of shame that they feel dependent on their partner whose love they desperately want. This may lead them to fear that they may become terribly ill if they leave on a business trip; in this situation, it feels more comfortable to worry about being ill than to acknowledge feeling so dependent and unable to function autonomously. Given an understanding of normal development, under more typical non-disaster situations, it is normal to develop a general sense that the world is a relatively-safe place and those who are responsible for one's welfare in fact have one's best interests in mind. Drastic deviations from this way of functioning in the absence of external catastrophe can provide clues that there was likely an early sense of insecurity and an internalized lack of trust, generated either systemically from the environment [59], or within the context of early formative relationships.

4 Psychodynamic Treatment of Separation Anxiety

Psychodynamic therapy takes advantage of the unique circumstance of the therapeutic space, and the developing therapeutic relationship in treating separation anxiety. It is within the relationship with the therapist, through a process of understanding and reflecting on feelings and actions, that patient and therapist can explore the conscious and unconscious forces at play underlying separation anxiety. Given the relational centrality of separation anxiety, the relationship that the separation anxious patient develops with the therapist serves as a guidepost, or *in vivo* laboratory, through which to explore key fantasies leading to symptoms. Links are made between what is happening in the room between the patient and therapist with what is taking place outside the room, in the context of separation anxious attachment relationships. The therapist tracks and helps the patient to explore the patient's emotional responses to missed sessions, vacations, and variations in schedule that can highlight feelings that arise with the therapist in the therapy. Even if no problems appear to be taking place in the therapeutic relationship, and if the patient appears improved from therapy, the relationship and underlying feelings should be explored, as in: why does the person feel they have improved? What might have served to calm the person down? The therapeutic relationship, with its underlying fantasies, called the "transference" is an emotionally vibrant paradigm through which to explore and intervene in this disorder [60].

In general, psychodynamic treatments share a number of core elements that arise from the generally accepted understanding that behavior and thinking emerge out of the human process of symbolizing conflicted emotional states. Manualized psychodynamic treatments progress through phases of elucidation of conflicts, working through and re-experiencing of core relational (attachment) themes in the therapeutic relationship (transference), and termination in which separation and individuation (development of a greater sense of autonomy) is explored directly. We have articulated these core components in our Child and Adolescent Anxiety Psychodynamic Psychotherapy (CAPP) [61] treatment manual.

The initial stage of psychodynamic psychotherapy for separation anxiety begins with the development of the relationship between patient and therapist and focuses on the elucidation of symptoms and their connection with the unconscious conflicts that underlie them, such as the conflicted and seemingly dangerous (i.e., potentially threatening in the context of the relationship with mother) wish to grow up and be a capable adult, while at the same time wanting to remain small and be cared for. Conflicts such as this are at the core of many fantasies, symptoms, and behaviors that constitute the syndromal presentation of separation anxiety, such as the feeling that going to school is frightening or the idea that one is too small, and doesn't really need to go to school. In patients with separation anxiety of all ages separating from central attachment figures is fraught with very mixed feelings. Patients wind up avoiding activities and situations that require separations in order to avoid facing these conflicts. Thus, separation anxiety often arises in the context of highly anxious, separation anxious families that are distressed by separations, which furthers patients' comfort with avoidance and limitations on autonomy. Entry into therapy may be one of the most separate activities the child or adult engages in, and being in treatment for separation anxiety can be felt as an unwelcome challenge to the apparent safety of enmeshment [60]. For these reasons, it is crucial to engage parents at least in the initial stages of the treatment of separation anxiety in children.

As treatment progresses and therapist and patient are more aware of the underlying conflicts, these conflicts generally emerge more clearly in the transference where these aspects of early attachments can begin to be articulated in language (rather than in the language of symptoms, action, and the body) between patient and therapist allowing for unconscious conflicts and conscious behaviors and understanding to take place. The patient generally becomes increasingly comfortable expressing their difficult emotions, such as rage at their controlling and anxious parent, which may first be experienced as feelings felt toward the therapist [60, 61]. The fantasy that these feelings are dangerous and might harm the patient themself, or those they love can be experienced and expressed in words in the treatment where they can be observed and tolerated together.

The final stage of dynamic therapy is termination, which is a particularly sensitive time for patients with separation anxiety as they are now forced to experience their fear of loss of an important attachment figure, and the need to internalize strengths they have developed and function more autonomously. This may be felt even more acutely by a patient who enters treatment after having experienced a real loss, such as the death of a parent. Termination in psychotherapy allows for very direct exploration of the feelings and thoughts that emerge in relationship to separation and loss.

Clinical Example

Blanca, a 38-year-old married mother of a 10-year-old presented with profound anxiety, panic attacks, and depression that were exacerbated every time her husband deviated from his work routine schedule. While her symptoms were global, they were driven by her profound separation anxiety. Victor, Blanca's husband, worked at the post office Tuesdays through Saturdays from 7 am until 4 pm, which meant that on days when he went to work and came home right afterward, he was available to help Blanca shop, cook, and help their son Brandon with his math homework. On days like these, Blanca reported that "I can just manage to survive," however, on the-relatively frequent- occasions that Victor took his ailing mother to the doctor, or devoted time to projects he cared about at their church, or chose to see friends, Blanca became overwhelmingly anxious and terrified that either he (more commonly) or she would die. Her symptoms became severe enough that she wound up vomiting, believing herself to have severe food poisoning or to be dying. Nothing helped other than Victor's breaking off other activities to race home and care for her. Tensions understandably mounted. Blanca's anxiety had been escalating, with frequent breakthroughs in severe anxiety and panic and thoughts of suicide ever since Victor had gone through an extensive job search and interviewing process for a position that would require him to travel for several days on a quarterly basis. Blanca had been in pharmacological treatment for her depression and anxiety for the past 9 years, and had completed several courses of CBT and exposure therapy with little improvement. In psychotherapy, it rapidly emerged that Blanca was in a state of nearly continuous rage at Victor. Even though she said many angry things about him while she reported her anxiety and her terror of "losing him," she seemed unaware that she felt this way. For example, she said: "Like I get terrified when he has to move the car at night. And he goes to do it, and I'm thinking-the thugs should get him, he's such a jerk. Then I'm mortified and I think God is going to hear me and punish me for this, he's going to die." So convinced did Blanca become that Victor's death was imminent that she would startle when he returned home after moving the car; in her mind she had already been planning his funeral. Gradually in therapy, the therapist was able to demonstrate to Blanca that she was having very violent thoughts toward Victor, reflecting longstanding rage and disappointments she had in the relationship, and she was living her life as though the vengeful, angry thoughts would come true every minute. Blanca's anxiety, depression, and severe separation anxiety improved as she began to recognize and acknowledge her fury at Victor for limiting her life in a number of crucial ways, from her perspective. Only once her rage became detoxified was Blanca able to take simple concrete steps that would bolster her own autonomy, such as finally getting a drivers' license. Blanca's separation anxiety, depression and panic attacks remitted after 3 months of psychotherapy [62].

References

1. Kessler RC, Berglund P, Demler O, Jin R, Merikangas KR, Walters EE. Lifetime prevalence and age of onset distributions of DSM IV disorders in the National Comorbidity Survey Replication. Arch Gen Psychiatry. 2005;62:593–602. Published erratum appears in Arch Gen Psychiatry, 62: 768.
2. Dell'Osso L, Carmassi C, Musetti L, Socci C, Shear MK, Conversano C, Maremmani II, Perugi G. Lifetime mood symptoms and adult separation anxiety in patients with complicated grief and/or post-traumatic stress disorder: a preliminary report. Psychiatry Res. 2012;198(3):436–40.
3. Pini S, Abelli M, Shear KM, Cardini A, Lar L, Gesi C, Muti M, Calugi S, Galderisi S, Troisi A, Bertolino A, Cassano GB. Frequency and clinical correlates of adult separation anxiety in a sample of 508 outpatients with mood and anxiety disorders. Acta Psychiatr Scand. 2010;122(1):40–6.
4. Ozten E, Tufan A, Eryilmaz G, Sayar G, Bulut H. The prevalence of adult separation anxiety disorder in a clinical sample of patients with ADHD. Anadolu Psikiyatri Dergisi. 2016;17(6):459.
5. Bowlby J. Separation anxiety: a critical review of the literature. J Child Psychol Psychiatry. 1960;1:231–26.
6. Mahler MS. On human symbiosis and the vicissitudes of individuation, Infantile psychosis, vol. 1. London: New York International Universities Press, Hogarth; 1968.
7. Bowlby J. Attachment and Loss. New York: Basic Books; 1973.
8. Bowlby J. A secure base: parent-child attachment and healthy human development. London: Routledge; 1988.
9. Freud S. Analysis of a phobia in a five-year-old boy (1909). In: Complete psychological works, standard ed, 10. London: Hogarth Press; 1955.
10. Milrod B, Markowitz JC, Gerber AJ, Cyranowski J, Altemus M, Shapiro T, Hofer M, Glatt C. Childhood separation anxiety and the pathogenesis and treatment of adult anxiety. Am J Psychiatr. 2014;171:34–43.

11. Winnicott D. The maturational processes and the facilitation environment. London: Hogarth Press; 1965.
12. Ainsworth MDS, Bell SM. Attachment, exploration and separation: illustrated by the behavior of one year olds in a strange situation. Child Dev. 1970;41:49–67.
13. Beebe B, Jaffe MS, Buck K, Chen H, Cohen P, Bahrick L, Andrews H, Feldstein S. The origins of 12-month attachment: a microanalysis of 4-month mother-infant interaction. Attach Hum Dev. 2010;12:3–141. https://doi.org/10.1080/14616730903338985.
14. Hofer M. Hidden regulators in attachment, separation and loss. Monographs Soc Res Child Dev. 1994;59:192–207.
15. Lyons-Ruth K, Block D. The disturbed caregiving system: relations among childhood trauma, maternal caregiving, and infant affect and attachment. Infant Ment Health J. 1996;17:257–75.
16. Feinman S, Roberts D, Hsieh KF, Sawyer D, Swanson D. A Critical review of social referencing in infancy. In: Feinman S, editor. Social referencing and the social construction of reality in infancy. Boston, MA: Springer; 1992. https://doi.org/10.1007/978-1-4899-2462-9_2.
17. Möller EL, Majdandžić M, Bögels SM. Fathers' versus mothers' social referencing signals in relation to infant anxiety and avoidance: a visual cliff experiment. Dev Sci. 2014;17(6):1012–28. https://doi.org/10.1111/desc.12194. Epub 2014 Jun 9. PMID: 24909521.
18. Sorce JF, Emde RN, Campos JJ, Klinnert MD. Maternal emotional signaling: its effect on the visual cliff behavior of 1-year-olds. Dev Psychol. 1985;21:195–200. https://doi.org/10.1037/0012-1649.21.1.195.
19. Spitz R. Hospitalism: an inquiry into the genesis of psychiatric conditions in early childhood. Psychoanal Study Child. 1945;1(1):53–74.
20. Spitz R. Anaclitic depression. Psychoanal Study Child. 1946;2(1):313–42.
21. Laor N, Wolmer L, Mayes LC, Golomb A, Silverberg DS, Weizman R, Cohen DJ. Israeli preschoolers under Scud missile attacks: a developmental perspective on risk-modifying factors. Arch Gen Psychiatry. 1996;53:416–23.
22. Chu AT, Lieberman AF. Clinical implications of traumatic stress from birth to age five. Annu Rev Clin Psychol. 2010;6:469–94.
23. Lieberman AF. Infants remember: war exposure, trauma, and attachment in young children and their mothers. J Am Acad Child Adolesc Psychiatry. 2011;50(7):640–1.
24. Borelli JL, Lai J, Smiley PA, Kerr ML, Buttitta K, Hecht HK, Rasmussen HF. Higher maternal reflective functioning is associated with toddlers' adaptive emotion regulation. Infant Ment Health J. 2020;42(4):473–87. https://doi.org/10.1002/imhj.21904.
25. Lund BL. Father– and mother–infant face-to-face interactions: differences in mind-related comments and infant attachment? Infant Behav Dev. 2003;26(2):200–12. Elsevier Inc, New York
26. Halfon S, Bekar O, Gürleyen BH, Mark J. An empirical analysis of mental state talk and affect regulation in two single-cases of psychodynamic child therapy. Psychotherapy (Chic). 2017;54(2):207–19.
27. Lowell AF, Peacock-Chambers E, Zayde A, DeCoste CL, McMahon TJ, Suchman NT. Mothering from the Inside out: addressing the intersection of addiction, adversity, and attachment with evidence-based parenting intervention. Curr Addict Rep. 2021;15:1–11. https://doi.org/10.1007/s40429-021-00389-1.
28. Suchman NE, DeCoste C, Borelli JL, McMahon TJ. Does improvement in maternal attachment representations predict greater maternal sensitivity, child attachment security and lower rates of relapse to substance use? A second test of Mothering from the Inside Out treatment mechanisms. J Subst Abuse Treat. 2018;85:21–30. https://doi.org/10.1016/j.jsat.2017.11.006.
29. Goodman G. The internal world and attachment. Hillsdale: Analytic Press; 2002.
30. Sandler J, Sandler AM. Internal objects revisited. London: Karnac; 1998.
31. Brunelli SA, Hofer MA. Selective breeding for infant rat separation-induced ultrasonic vocalizations: developmental precursors of passive and active coping styles. Behav Brain Res. 2007;182:193–207.
32. Hofer MA. Multiple regulators of ultrasonic vocalization in the infant rat. Psychoneuroendocrinology. 1996;21:203–17.

33. Coplan JD, Mathew SJ, Abdallah CG, Mao X, Kral JG, Smith EL, Rosenblum LA, Perera TD, Dwork AJ, Hof PR, Gorman JM, Shungu DC. Early-life stress and neurometabolites of the hippocampus. Brain Res. 2010;1358:191–9.
34. Coplan JD, Abdallah CG, Kaufman J, Gelernter J, Smith EL, Perera TD, Dwork AJ, Kaffman A, Gorman JM, Rosenblum LA, Owens MJ, Nemeroff CB. Early-life stress, corticotropin-releasing factor, and serotonin transporter gene: a pilot study. Psychoneuroendocrinology. 2011;36:289–93.
35. Jackowski A, Perera TD, Abdallah CG, Garrido G, Tang CY, Martinez J, Mathew SJ, Gorman JM, Rosenblum LA, Smith EL, Dwork AJ, Shungu DC, Kaffman A, Gelernter J, Coplan JD, Kaufman J. Early-life stress, corpus callosum development, hippocampal volumetrics, and anxious behavior in male nonhuman primates. Psychiatry Res. 2011;192(1):37–44. https://doi.org/10.1016/j.pscychresns.2010.11.006. Epub 2011 Mar 5. PMID: 21377844; PMCID: PMC4090111.
36. Eapen V, Dadds M, Barnett B, Kohlhoff J, Khan F, Radom N, Silove DM. Separation anxiety, attachment and inter-personal representations: disentangling the role of oxytocin in the perinatal period. PLoS One. 2014;9(9):e107745.
37. Mahler MS. A study of the separation individuation process with possible application to borderline phenomena in the psychoanalytic situation. Psychoanal Study Child. 1971;26:403–24.
38. Mahler MS. On the first three subphases of the separation-individuation process. Int J Psychoanal. 1972;53:333–8.
39. Beebe B, Lachmann FM, Jaffe J. A transformational model of presymbolic representations. Psychoanal Dial. 1997;7(2):207–13.
40. Beebe B, Lachmann FM. Chapter 1 mother—infant mutual influence and precursors of psychic structure. Progr Self Psychol. 1988;3:3–25.
41. Fonagy P. Can we use observations of infant-caregiver interactions as the basis for a model of the representational world? Psychoanal Dial. 1997;7(2):207–13.
42. Carlson EA, Egeland B, Sroufe V. A prospective investigation of the development of borderline personality symptoms. Dev Psychopathol. 1993;21(4):1311–13341.
43. Suess GJ, Grossmann KE, Sroufe LA. Effects of infant attachment to mother and father on quality of adaptation in preschool: from dyadic to individual organisation of self. Int J Behav Dev. 1992;15(1):43–65.
44. Main M, Solomon J. Discovery of an insecure-disorganized/disoriented attachment pattern. In: Brazelton TB, Yogman MW, editors. Affective development in infancy. New York: Ablex Publishing; 1986. p. 95–124.
45. Shah PE, Fonagy P, Strathearn L. Is attachment transmitted across generations? The plot thickens. Clin Child Psychol Psychiatry. 2010;15(3):329–45.
46. Main M, Goldwyn R. Adult attachment scoring and classification system. Unpublished scoring manual. Department of Psychology, University of California, Berkeley, 1985–1994.
47. Last CG, Hersen M, Kazdin AE, Francis G, Grubb HJ. Psychiatric illness in the mothers of anxious children. Am J Psychiatry. 1987;144:1580–3.
48. Biederman J, Rosenbaum JF, Bolduc-Murphy EA, Faraone SV, Chaloff J, Hirshfeld DR, Kagan J. A 3-year follow-up of children with and without behavioral inhibition. J Am Acad Child Adolesc Psychiatry. 1993;32(4):814–21.
49. Hirshfeld-Becker DR, Biederman J, Henin A, Faraone SV, Davis S, Harrington K, Rosenbaum JF. Behavioral inhibition in preschool children at risk is a specific predictor of middle childhood social anxiety: a five-year follow-up. J Dev Behav Pediatr. 2007;28(3):225–33.
50. Hirshfeld-Becker DR, Micco J, Henin A, Bloomfield A, Biederman J, Rosenbaum J. Behavioral inhibition. Depress Anxiety. 2008;25:357–67.
51. Suomi SJ. Early determinants of behaviour: evidence from primate studies. Br Med Bull. 1997;53:170–84.
52. Maag B, Phelps PA, Kiel EJ. Do maternal parenting behaviors indirectly link toddler dysregulated fear and child anxiety symptoms? Child Psychiatry Hum Dev. 2020;52(2):225–35. https://doi.org/10.1007/s10578-020-01004-6.

53. Kagan J, Reznick JS, Snidman N. Biological bases of childhood shyness. Science. 1988;240:167–71.
54. Orgiles M, Penosa P, Morales A, Fernandez-Martinez I, Espada J. Maternal anxiety and separation anxiety in children aged between 3 and 6 years mediating role of parenting style. J Dev Behav Pediatrics. 2018;39:621–8.
55. Battaglia M, Pesenti-Gritti P, Medland SE, Ogliari A, Tambs K, Spatola CAM. A genetically informed study of the association between childhood separation anxiety, sensitivity to CO_2, panic disorder, and the effect of childhood parental loss. Arch Gen Psychiatry. 2009;66(1):64–71. https://doi.org/10.1001/archgenpsychiatry:513.
56. Ehrenreich JT, Santucci LC, Weiner CL. Separation anxiety disorder in youth: phenomenology, assessment, and treatment. Psicol Conductual. 2008;16(3):389–412. https://doi.org/10.1901/jaba.2008.16-389.
57. Sirin HD. Parental acceptance-rejection and adult separation anxiety: the mediation of adult attachment insecurity. SAGE Open. 2019;9(4):215824401988513. https://doi.org/10.1177/2158244019885138.
58. Tennes KH, Lampl EE. Defensive reactions to infantile separation anxiety. J Am Psychoanal Assoc. 1969;17:1142–62.
59. Baldwin J. The fire next time. New York: Vintage International; 1963.
60. Preter S, Shapiro T, Milrod B. Child and adolescent anxiety psychodynamic psychotherapy: a manual. Oxford: Oxford University Press; 2018. Print ISBN-13:9780190877712
61. Milrod B, Shapiro S, Gross C, Silver G, Preter S, Libow A, Leon AC. Does manualized psychodynamic psychotherapy have an impact on youth anxiety disorders? Am J Psychother. 2013;67:359–66.
62. Busch F, Milrod B, Singer M, Aronson A. Panic focused psychodynamic psychotherapy: eXtended range: psychodynamic psychotherapy for anxiety disorders: a transdiagnostic treatment manual. Milton Park: Taylor & Francis, LLC.; 2012.

Separation Anxiety in the DSM-5

Jill M. Cyranowski

Prior to the DSM-5, separation anxiety disorder was relegated to the DSM-IV section devoted to "Disorders Usually First Diagnosed in Infancy, Childhood, or Adolescence." Thus, it comes as little surprise that this DSM diagnosis has historically been considered a disorder of early childhood by clinical practitioners. Indeed, the DSM-IV-TR guidebook [1] explicitly instructed that "only rarely is it appropriate to make this diagnosis in adults" (p. 390) and even then the diagnosis could only be applied to adults in cases where there was sufficient evidence to support symptom onset prior to age 18. It was only with the advent of the DSM-5 that separation anxiety disorder was moved to reside with other anxiety disorders as part of the manual's "Anxiety Disorders" section, with explicit wording that allowed the diagnosis to be made across the developmental spectrum, regardless of the individual's current age or age of symptom onset [2, 3].

In the following chapter, we review the developmental origins of the separation anxiety construct, and its initial operationalization as a childhood disorder. We then discuss burgeoning evidence regarding the prevalence and effective measurement of this construct in both pediatric and adult populations, including research to support the impairing nature of this disorder in adults. We review data available on the course and common comorbidities related to this diagnosis, as well as factors that may contribute to continued under-diagnosis of adult separation anxiety. Finally, we discuss preliminary work to incorporate the measurement of separation insecurity within the HiTOP (Hierarchical Taxonomy of Psychopathology) model, as well as future psychometric and clinical work needed for the field to fully embrace separation anxiety disorder as a diagnostic entity that can impact both pediatric and adult populations.

J. M. Cyranowski (✉)
Department of Psychology, University of Pittsburgh, Pittsburgh, PA, USA
e-mail: jcyranow@pitt.edu

S. Pini, B. Milrod (eds.), *Separation Anxiety in Adulthood*,
https://doi.org/10.1007/978-3-031-37446-3_4

1 Origins of the Childhood Separation Anxiety Disorder Construct

The diagnosis of separation anxiety disorder has its roots in both developmental research and attachment theory. Distress in response to separation from a primary caregiver, often in the form of one's mother, represents a developmental norm during early childhood [4–7]. Indeed, the experience and expression of separation distress in young children has been theorized to carry adaptive evolutionary value, by helping the defenseless offspring to maintain close proximity to primary caregivers on whom they rely for both safety and sustenance [5, 6]. Early attachment relationships with responsive primary caregivers has been postulated to promote the development of mental schemas of oneself and others that support the ability to utilize primary caregivers as a "secure base" from which one can confidently explore one's environment while knowing that primary attachment figures will be consistently available for support in times of stress or need [4, 5]. Thus, early infant–caregiver interactions foster social bonding and the development of secure attachment representations (including the view of oneself as lovable and others as caring and available), which are carried into adolescent and adult relationships [8, 9]. Secure attachment patterns, in turn, facilitate the development, maintenance, and effective utilization of supportive social relationships in ways that allow the individual to develop independent mastery and self-efficacy while maintaining a sense of confidence that close attachment figures will be available and responsive in times of need.

Observational studies of infants and toddlers confirm the normative expressions of distress upon separation from one's mother or the introduction of an unknown stranger or situation [10]. Normal expressions of separation distress can appear as early as 4 months of age, often peaking between 13 and 18 months [11]. Some levels of separation discomfort or distress are also common across early childhood, and are not atypical as children leave their home environments to begin daycare, school or peer social activities. Thus, it is only when expressions of separation distress become *excessive, prolonged, developmentally inappropriate or impairing* that a diagnosis of separation anxiety disorder would be considered. Given these diagnostic considerations, it is perhaps unsurprising that childhood separation anxiety disorder is often first identified when school-age children are unable to effectively separate from parental figures and present with persistent somatic symptoms (such as chronic abdominal pain) which often arise in the context of school refusal behaviors [12].

Included in the third iteration of the DSM and beyond, the diagnostic criteria for separation anxiety disorder are centered on excessive, developmentally inappropriate anxiety related to perceived or anticipated separation from primary attachment figures. Current diagnosis of separation anxiety disorder in the DSM-5 requires that patients meet at least three of eight Category A criteria, including: excessive distress when faced with actual or anticipated separation from home or primary attachment figures; refusal or significant reluctance to leave home or go out because of separation fears; fears of being alone (without attachment figures) at home or in other settings; refusal or significant reluctance to sleep away from home or attachment figures; worries about losing or harm befalling attachment figures (i.e., via injury, illness or death); worries about experiencing an untoward event that would cause one to be separated from attachment figures (like being kidnapped, lost, or in an accident); repeated nightmares that relate to themes of separation from attachment figures; and significant physical symptoms or complaints (such as stomachaches, nausea, headaches) in the face of actual or anticipated separation [3].

The core concepts included in these separation anxiety disorder criteria have been relatively stable across versions of the DSM. On a conceptual level, the criteria are not themselves age limited. However, text descriptions of these diagnoses up through DSM-IV-R utilized language and examples that were clearly child-oriented. For example, the third and fourth editions of the DSM discussed examples of clinging behaviors, shadowing parents around the house, fears of monsters and the dark, difficulties with separation at bedtime, sleep-overs and summer camps, and school refusal behaviors. Moreover, discussion of diagnostic differentials primarily focused on other childhood phenomenon or disorders, such as developmentally appropriate separation anxiety in children, overanxious disorder (in the DSM-III and DSM-III-R), conduct disorder, and pervasive developmental disorders. Thus, despite the fact that a diagnosis of separation anxiety disorder could technically be made in an adult using the DSM-IV-R criteria, the diagnostic description itself was heavily focused on the experience of separation anxiety in childhood, and the diagnosis required that an adult being considered for the diagnosis retrospectively report symptom onset prior to age 18.

2 Expanding the Reach of the Separation Anxiety Construct into Adulthood

Despite early accounts and diagnostic criteria that painted separation anxiety as a disorder specific to childhood, the 1990s saw the emergence of research supporting the existence, potential measurement, and prevalence of adult variants of this disorder. Among some of the earliest clinical researchers to focus on adult separation anxiety, Silove, Manicavasagar, and colleagues posited the clinical importance of this construct and developed self-report scales to assess not only adults' retrospective accounts of childhood separation anxiety [utilizing the *Separation Anxiety Symptom Inventory* or SASI [13]], but also core symptoms of separation anxiety as experienced throughout adulthood [utilizing the *Adult Separation Anxiety Structured Interview* (ASA-SI) or self-report checklist (ASA-27) [14, 15]]. These authors speculated that the core features of separation anxiety disorder—namely excessive levels of anxiety and often disabling distress when faced with perceived or anticipated separation from major attachment figures—may persist and/or arise de novo in adulthood [14, 16–18]. Thus, the authors' 27-item adult separation anxiety checklist articulated facets of separation anxiety from an adult perspective. This scale includes age-appropriate manifestations of characteristic separation anxiety symptoms that may be experienced in the context of adult relationships, such as separation fears, physical symptoms, and nightmares or avoidance of being alone or apart from close relationship partners. In addition, this scale includes uniquely adult manifestations of separation anxiety that have been observed in clinical practice, such as concerns about the intensity or closeness of relationships; the experience of worrying about where significant others are, what they are doing, or needing to call often to check in on them; excessive distress when needing to travel, sleep apart or change daily routines that ensure close contact with attachment figures; or even finding that one talks excessively in order to maintain contact with close relationship partners [14, 19]. The ASA-27 self-report scale has been shown to display good internal consistency [with Cronbach's alphas ranging from 0.85 to 0.95 [14, 19, 20]], sound test-retest reliability [r = 0.86 over an average 3-week period [15]], and concurrent validity with interview-based clinical assessments of adult separation anxiety [14, 15, 19, 20]

Building on the need to develop psychometrically-sound diagnostic assessments of separation anxiety disorder in adults, Shear and colleagues developed a structured clinical interview to assess each of the eight DSM-IV separation anxiety disorder criteria utilizing age-appropriate child and adult descriptions [20, 21]. This instrument, termed the *Structured Clinical Interview for Separation Anxiety Symptoms* or SCI-SAS, was developed for use in adults. This structured interview includes two 8-item scales that separately assess childhood experiences of separation anxiety (using retrospective recall of experiences prior to age 18) and age-appropriate adult separation anxiety, both based on DSM diagnostic criteria. Each criterion is scored by the clinical interviewer as 0 (not at all), 1 (sometimes), 2 (often) or? (don't recall). In keeping with DSM diagnostic standards, endorsement of three or more of the eight symptoms at a threshold score of 2 (often) is needed to make a categorical diagnosis of separation anxiety disorder in childhood and adulthood. Moreover, summing all symptoms, including those rated at a subthreshold (1—sometimes) level allows for a continuous rating of the severity of separation anxiety symptoms experienced during childhood and adulthood. These scales have been shown to have good internal consistency, with Cronbach's alphas of 0.79 for the child scale and 0.85 for the adult scale [20]. While both scales appear to tap a core, underlying separation anxiety construct, factor analytic work indicate that the two child-focused criteria that include explicit reference to school refusal behaviors (i.e., reluctance or refusal to go out and specifically to school, and physical symptoms when faced with anticipated separation, such as going to school) appeared to be related to, but distinguishable from, the primary child separation anxiety disorder construct. This likely points to the fact that during childhood, school refusal behaviors may occur for a variety of reasons, only one of which may relate to the experience of childhood separation anxiety.

Notably, the SCI-SAS child and adult clinical interview scales also show predictable patterns of multi-trait, multi-method convergent, and discriminant validity when assessed alongside other interview and self-report scales. Specifically, the interview-based child and adult SCI-SAS scales showed unique and strong patterns of correlation with the above-mentioned child [13] and adult [14] separation anxiety self-report scales (r's = 0.85 and 0.84 for the SASI and ASA-27 scales, respectively). In contrast, the scales displayed significant yet weaker associations with clinical interview and self-report measures of panic disorder (with r's ranging from 0.46 to 0.57). Finally, scores on the child and adult SCI-SAS scales were moderately correlated ($r = 0.66$), yet clearly not redundant with one another [20].

3 Diagnostic Epidemiology of Separation Anxiety Disorder

Inclusion of structured interview questions resembling the SCI-SAS within the National Comorbidity Survey Replication (NCS-R) for the DSM-IV, which studied 5692 adults in the USA, provided initial lifetime prevalence rates of 4.1% for retrospectively reported childhood separation anxiety disorder, and 6.6% for adult separation anxiety disorder [21]. Notably, among adults who retrospectively reported experiencing childhood separation anxiety disorder, only about one-third (36.1%) endorsed syndromal separation anxiety symptoms that persisted into adulthood. Supporting the idea that separation anxiety may arise de novo in adulthood, three-quarters (77.5%) of respondents endorsing adult separation anxiety disorder reported first onset in adulthood [21]. Additional analyses that combined both adult (NCS-R) and adolescent data [from the NCS Adolescent Supplement or NCS-A, which included adolescents aged 13–17 [22]] obtained an even higher lifetime separation anxiety disorder prevalence rate of 7.7% for adolescents aged 13–17, and an overall lifetime morbid risk rate (an estimate of the proportion of people who will develop separation anxiety disorder at some point in their lives) of 8.7% among US samples aged 13 and over [23]. Data from the combined NCS-R/NCS-A report also provided 12-month separation anxiety disorder prevalence at 1.2% in US samples aged 13 and up [23].

Looking at epidemiologic data worldwide, Silove et al. have reported lifetime separation anxiety disorder prevalence rates of 4.8% and 12-month prevalence rates of 1.0% in a World Health Organization (WHO) sample of 38,993 adults spanning 18 countries [24], assessed using the WHO Composite International Diagnostic Interview (CIDI). Supporting previous work by Shear et al. [21] with respect to the existence of adult-onset separation anxiety disorder, Silove and colleagues reported that a full 43.1% of adults endorsing lifetime separation anxiety disorder indicated that first onset occurred in adulthood [24]. In additional analyses controlling for country, age, and comorbid lifetime disorders, Silove and colleagues found that the experience of maladaptive family functioning in childhood (as indicated by such factors as parental mental illness or substance abuse, domestic violence or child abuse), other childhood adversities (such as parental illness, death, divorce, extended separation from a parent, or economic adversity), other lifetime traumas (such as the experience of natural disaster, war, or violence), and female gender predicted diagnosis of lifetime separation anxiety disorder.

In their WHO study, Silove et al. found that lifetime prevalence rates of separation anxiety disorder were higher for women in 15 of the 18 countries studied, with the combined sample providing an estimate of lifetime prevalence rates of 5.6% and 4.0% in women and men, respectively [24]. These gender differences parallel findings of higher rates of lifetime separation anxiety disorder in females relative to males within US epidemiologic data sets. Specifically, Kessler et al. reported lifetime prevalence rates of separation anxiety disorder among samples aged 13 and up (including the NCS-R and NCS-A data sets) of 8.3% for women and 5.2% for males [23]. There are, however, some data to suggest that gender differences in separation anxiety disorder diagnoses may be more pronounced in child versus adult samples. For example, using the adult NCS-R sample, Shear et al. reported female:male odds ratios of 2.2 for separation anxiety disorder reported during childhood, and 1.4 for separation anxiety disorder reported in adulthood [21].

Both current and lifetime rates of separation anxiety disorder have been shown to be considerably higher within adult clinical samples. For example, in one sample of 508 psychiatric outpatients treated for mood and anxiety disorders in adult psychiatric outpatient clinics in Italy, Pini et al. found that a full 50.8% reported a lifetime history of separation anxiety disorder, including 8.5% who endorsed childhood separation anxiety only, 21.7% who reported a history of both childhood and adult separation anxiety, and 20.75% who reported a history of adult separation anxiety disorder only [25]. Similarly, in a sample of 520 adults presenting to an anxiety disorder outpatient clinic in Australia, Silove and colleagues estimated that when a diagnosis of adult separation anxiety disorder was considered, it would have comprised 23% of all current diagnoses made (including both primary and comorbid diagnoses) [26].

Further supporting the diagnostic utility of the adult separation anxiety disorder construct, multiple studies support the high level of role impairment associated with this diagnosis. Within the USA, NCS-R data indicate that among adults endorsing separation anxiety disorder in the past 12 months, more than 40% report severe impairment in at least one domain of the Sheehan Disability Scale [21], with the most severe impairments occurring within social and personal domains of function. To account for the high rates of mood and anxiety disorder comorbidity and their impacts on function, Shear et al. [21] also separately evaluated those respondents endorsing 12-month separation anxiety disorder without any other 12-month mood or anxiety disorder—which they classified as "pure 12-month separation anxiety disorder." Notably, these analyses indicated that among those individuals meeting criteria for "pure 12-month separation anxiety disorder," 63.2% reported some level of functional impairment, with 29.8% reporting severe impairment [21]. As part of the cross-national WHO study, Silove et al. [24] similarly found that a full 42.4% of individuals endorsing 12-month separation anxiety disorder reported severe levels of role impairment, utilizing a modified version of the Sheehan Disability Scale [24]. Research evaluating clinical samples of mood and anxiety disorder patients further support the incremental impact of separation anxiety disorder on various aspects of life functioning. For example, among Pini et al.'s sample of 508 outpatients with mood and anxiety disorders, patients with adult separation anxiety disorder were shown to report greater role impairment in occupational and relationship function on the Sheehan Disability Scale, as compared with psychiatric outpatients without adult separation anxiety disorder, even after statistically controlling for psychiatric comorbidities and gender [25].

4 Separation Anxiety Disorder Course and Comorbidities

Among the childhood anxiety disorders, separation anxiety disorder has long been considered one of the most prevalent and earliest to emerge, with onset commonly reported between 7 and 12 years in child clinical samples [27–29]. Similarly, in the Shear et al. [21] report, the age of disorder onset for adults retrospectively reporting childhood separation anxiety disorder fell in early to middle childhood. In contrast, individuals reporting adult-onset separation anxiety disorder reported disorder onset in the late teens to early 20s, with a full 80% reporting first onset prior to age 30 [21]. Thus, it is not surprising that retrospective age of onset reports among US epidemiologic samples (aged 13 and up) that consider the potential for either childhood or adult separation anxiety disorder onset estimate median age of onset between 15 and 17 years, and continue to identify separation anxiety disorder (along with phobias) as the earliest to emerge across the mood and anxiety disorders [23].

Given the early age of onset of separation anxiety disorder and the high comorbidity rates observed among separation anxiety and other anxiety and mood disorders, many have theorized regarding etiologic or shared pathophysiologic mechanisms. Based on his early observation that many adult patients suffering from panic attacks retrospectively reported symptoms of childhood separation anxiety, Klein hypothesized that panic may specifically relate to early innate separation anxiety mechanisms [30]. Others have similarly posited specific links between childhood separation anxiety and later experience of panic or agoraphobia which may relate, in part, to similarities in symptom profiles. For example, periods of intense, acute distress that may become associated with somatic symptoms are common in both separation anxiety and panic. Similarly, symptoms of discomfort, fear or avoidance of leaving home or being without a close relationship partner (whose presence promotes a sense of safety) are common in both separation anxiety and agoraphobia.

While elevated reports of retrospectively-assessed childhood separation anxiety have been obtained in samples of adults with panic disorder, most data point to a more general link between childhood separation anxiety and a variety of adult mood and anxiety disorders [31]. For example, in one early study of 252 adults recruited from an anxiety disorder research clinic, Lipsitz et al. observed that patients who met DSM-III-R criteria for childhood separation anxiety disorder were more likely to meet criteria for two or more current, co-occurring anxiety disorders [32]. However, these researchers did not find a specific association between childhood separation anxiety and adult panic disorder per se.

The existence of separation anxiety disorder observed within clinical samples has, however, been associated with elevated levels of mood and anxiety symptoms more generally. For example, in one study of 235 outpatients with panic disorder, Gesi and colleagues found that 53.2% reported comorbid separation anxiety disorder, and that this diagnosis was associated with greater levels of panic, mood and manic/hypomanic symptoms (as well as a greater likelihood of being younger and female) [33]. Similarly, in a sample of 100 outpatients being treated for major depressive disorder, Elbay and colleagues observed that 41% also met criteria for adult separation anxiety, and that those with separation anxiety disorder comorbidity were more likely to display additional anxiety disorder comorbidities and to require treatment with newer generation antidepressants and other adjunctive medications [34]. Similarly, Pini and colleagues observed that outpatients with comorbid separation anxiety disorder reported a greater number of lifetime depressive episodes [25].

Initial data also suggest that separation anxiety disorder may constitute a risk factor for development of such stress-related disorders as complicated grief and PTSD. Shear et al. found that individuals whose childhood separation anxiety symptoms persisted into adulthood were at increased risk to experience complicated grief [35]. And in a study of refugees of war-torn Bosnia, half of those with PTSD were found to also meet criteria for adult separation anxiety disorder. Notably, however, almost all who met criteria for adult separation anxiety disorder in this traumatized population reported PTSD, which may speak to the psychopathology risk involved when individuals with underlying separation anxiety sensitivities experience intense stress, trauma or loss [36].

Taken together, these data suggest that individuals whose childhood separation anxiety persists into adulthood may be at particular risk of experiencing affective, anxiety and stress-related disorders in the face of future life stress. Such data speak to broader attachment theory models linking early insecure attachment patterns to risk of adult psychopathology [37–39]. Thus, early and persistent separation anxiety symptoms may represent a marker of underlying attachment insecurity—which may lead to both observed manifestations of separation sensitivity and distress, as well as risk for additional mood and anxiety pathology in the face of future life stress, trauma or loss [37, 39].

5 DSM-5 and Beyond: Diagnostic Differentials and Continuous Models of Psychopathology

A number of DSM anxiety and personality disorders share symptomatic features with separation anxiety disorder. This situation likely contributes to ongoing patterns of missed or mis-diagnosis with the DSM-5, particularly in adult clinical samples for whom separation anxiety pathology is often overlooked [2, 26]. As noted above, separation anxiety and panic disorder share features of acute distress and fear. Yet while individuals with separation anxiety may experience panic-like symptoms, the underlying fear is focused on separation from key attachment figures rather than fears of physiologic sensations, as seen in panic disorder. Similarly, while individuals with separation anxiety may restrict traveling from home that may appear, on the surface, similar to agoraphobia, the underlying fear is that an untoward event may lead to separation from attachment figures—and not agoraphobic fears of being in places where escape would be difficult or where obtaining help would be impossible. Symptoms of separation anxiety may similarly be misclassified as generalized anxiety disorder in adults [26]. Indeed, separation anxiety and GAD have previously been found to be particularly comorbid among child clinical samples [40]. Here, however, the diagnostic differential lies in the fact that worry about separation from key attachment figures (which may occur through a variety of untoward events) represents the primary worry in separation anxiety disorder, rather than being only one among a variety of differing concerns that alternate as the focus of worry as observed in generalized anxiety disorder.

Many authors have also noted diagnostic similarities between separation anxiety disorder and personality disorders such as borderline or dependent personality disorder. Data do suggest elevated levels of personality pathology in clinical samples of adults with separation anxiety, and particularly among those who report childhood onset of separation anxiety symptoms [41]. While borderline personality disorder may include fears of abandonment or frantic efforts to avoid abandonment (as may be seen in separation anxiety disorder), this is but one of many borderline symptoms including such features as identity disturbance, feelings of emptiness, unstable personal relationships, impulsivity, anger and affective instability, and suicidal or self-harm behaviors. Similarly, both separation anxiety disorder and dependent personality disorder share features related to the wish or need to keep attachment figures close at hand. However, dependent personality disorder is characterized by an over-reliance on other people more generally (often including key attachment figures as well as others in one's life) because of a lack of confidence in one's own self-efficacy and a perceived need for help with daily decision-making and reassurance-seeking. In contrast, separation anxiety disorder is more specifically focused on attempts to keep key attachment figures close out of fears for their safety and the potential for separation or loss [2].

Proponents of dimensional approaches to psychopathology assessment, including the Hierarchical Taxonomy of Psychopathology (HiTOP), point to the above-noted symptom overlap levels and the high comorbidity levels observed across DSM-5 diagnoses as evidence of the inherent problems of current categorical diagnostic approaches [42, 43]. In contrast to research based on traditional, clinically-derived categorical diagnoses, HiTOP proponents argue for an empirical, quantitative approach to nosology that seeks to uncover the underlying hierarchical structure and core subdomains of psychopathological symptoms. As part of this hierarchical model, the higher order *Internalizing Spectrum* includes component subfactors of symptom constellations including fear (that would include such DSM related disorders as panic and agoraphobia) and distress (that would include such DSM related disorders as GAD, MDD, and Borderline PD). In this vein, recent work to develop preliminary HiTOP internalizing spectrum scales have included a homogeneous composite scale of eight items related to "Separation Insecurity" which was found to load onto higher order dimensions of both Distress and Social/Somatic Anxiety [44]. Further work is needed, however, including work to better understand this "Separation Insecurity" symptom scale and its potential relationship to extant self-report and interview measures of separation anxiety as well as categorical DSM-5 Separation Anxiety Disorder diagnosis.

6 Conclusions and Future Research Directions

A significant body of research now supports the DSM-5 inclusion of separation anxiety disorder as an anxiety disorder with diagnostic and functional implications for both pediatric and adult populations [2]. Yet, despite research to support the measurement validity and debilitating nature of this diagnostic entity in adults, much work is needed to overcome the clinical perception of separation anxiety as a pediatric disorder, and to increase the field's identification, understanding, and treatment of separation anxiety disorder within adult populations. Because separation anxiety has only recently been included as an adult-appropriate diagnosis in the DSM-5, data are also needed to determine the longitudinal course of childhood separation anxiety in protocols that prospectively assess separation anxiety alongside other lifetime anxiety and mood disorders. Finally, future research to understand the underlying attachment-based dysfunction of separation anxiety disorder, its potential dimensional assessment, and its impact on risk for a variety of mood, anxiety, and stress-based disorders and symptom constellations is needed.

References

1. First MB, Frances A, Pincus HA. DSM-IV-TR guidebook. 1st ed. Washington, DC: American Psychiatric Pub.; 2004. p. xi. p 501
2. Bogels SM, Knappe S, Clark LA. Adult separation anxiety disorder in DSM-5. Clin Psychol Rev. 2013;33(5):663–74.
3. APA. Diagnostic and statistical manual of mental disorders, fifth edition (DSM-5). Washington, DC: American Psychiatric Publishing; 2013.
4. Ainsworth MD. The development of infant-mother interaction among the Ganda. In: Foss BM, editor. Determinants of infant behavior. New York: Wiley; 1963. p. 67–104.
5. Bowlby J. Attachment and loss, Attachment, vol. 1. New York: Basic Books; 1969.
6. Bowlby J. Attachment and loss, Separation: anxiety and anger, vol. 2. New York: Basic Books; 1973.
7. Bowlby J. A secure base: parent-child attachment and health human development. New York: Basic Books; 1988.
8. Collins NL, Read SJ. Adult attachment, working models, and relationship quality in dating couples. J Pers Soc Psychol. 1990;58(4):644–63.
9. Bartholomew K, Horowitz LM. Attachment styles among young adults: a test of a four-category model. J Pers Soc Psychol. 1991;61(2):226–44.
10. Ainsworth MD, Blehar MD, Waters E, Walls S. Patterns of attachment: a psychological study of the strange situation. Hillsdale, NJ: Erlbaum; 1978.
11. Emde RN, Gaensbauer TJ, Harmon RJ. Emotional expression in infancy; a biobehavioral study. Psychol Issues. 1976;10(01):1–200.
12. Masi G, Mucci M, Millepiedi S. Separation anxiety disorder in children and adolescents: epidemiology, diagnosis and management. CNS Drugs. 2001;15(2):93–104.
13. Silove D, Manicavasagar V, O'Connell D, Blaszczynski A, Wagner R, Henry J. The development of the Separation Anxiety Symptom Inventory (SASI). Aust N Z J Psychiatry. 1993;27(3):477–88.
14. Manicavasagar V, Silove D, Curtis J. Separation anxiety in adulthood: a phenomenological investigation. Compr Psychiatry. 1997;38(5):274–82.
15. Manicavasagar V, Silove D, Wagner R, Drobny J. A self-report questionnaire for measuring separation anxiety in adulthood. Compr Psychiatry. 2003;44(2):146–53.

16. Silove D, Manicavasagar V, Curtis J, Blaszczynski A. Is early separation anxiety a risk factor for adult panic disorder?: a critical review. Compr Psychiatry. 1996;37(3):167–79.
17. Manicavasagar V, Silove D. Is there an adult form of separation anxiety disorder? A brief clinical report. Aust N Z J Psychiatry. 1997;31(2):299–303.
18. Manicavasagar V, Silove D, Hadzi-Pavlovic D. Subpopulations of early separation anxiety: relevance to risk of adult anxiety disorders. J Affect Disord. 1998;48(2–3):181–90.
19. Manicavasagar V, Silove D, Curtis J, Wagner R. Continuities of separation anxiety from early life into adulthood. J Anxiety Disord. 2000;14(1):1–18.
20. Cyranowski JM, Shear MK, Rucci P, Fagiolini A, Frank E, Grochocinski VJ, et al. Adult separation anxiety: psychometric properties of a new structured clinical interview. J Psychiatr Res. 2002;36(2):77–86.
21. Shear K, Jin R, Ruscio AM, Walters EE, Kessler RC. Prevalence and correlates of estimated DSM-IV child and adult separation anxiety disorder in the National Comorbidity Survey Replication. Am J Psychiatry. 2006;163(6):1074–83.
22. Merikangas KR, Avenevoli S, Costello EJ, Koretz D, Kessler RC. National comorbidity survey replication adolescent supplement (NCS-A): I. Background and measures. J Am Acad Child Adolesc Psychiatry. 2009;48(4):367–79.
23. Kessler RC, Petukhova M, Sampson NA, Zaslavsky AM, Wittchen HU. Twelve-month and lifetime prevalence and lifetime morbid risk of anxiety and mood disorders in the United States. Int J Methods Psychiatr Res. 2012;21(3):169–84.
24. Silove D, Alonso J, Bromet E, Gruber M, Sampson N, Scott K, et al. Pediatric-onset and adult-onset separation anxiety disorder across countries in the world mental health survey. Am J Psychiatry. 2015;172(7):647–56.
25. Pini S, Abelli M, Shear KM, Cardini A, Lari L, Gesi C, et al. Frequency and clinical correlates of adult separation anxiety in a sample of 508 outpatients with mood and anxiety disorders. Acta Psychiatr Scand. 2010;122(1):40–6.
26. Silove DM, Marnane CL, Wagner R, Manicavasagar VL, Rees S. The prevalence and correlates of adult separation anxiety disorder in an anxiety clinic. BMC Psychiatry. 2010;10:21.
27. Keller MB, Lavori PW, Wunder J, Beardslee WR, Schwartz CE, Roth J. Chronic course of anxiety disorders in children and adolescents. J Am Acad Child Psychiatry. 1992;31(4):595–9.
28. Compton SN, Nelson AH, March JS. Social phobia and separation anxiety symptoms in community and clinical samples of children and adolescents. J Am Acad Child Psychiatry. 2000;39(8):1040–6.
29. Allen JL, Rapee RM, Sandberg S. Severe life events and chronic adversities as antecedents to anxiety in children: a matched control study. J Abnorm Child Psychol. 2008;36(7):1047–56.
30. Klein DF. False suffocation alarms, spontaneous panics, and related conditions. An integrative hypothesis. Arch Gen Psychiatry. 1993;50(4):306–17.
31. Kossowsky J, Pfaltz MC, Schneider S, Taeymans J, Locher C, Gaab J. The separation anxiety hypothesis of panic disorder revisited: a meta-analysis. Am J Psychiatry. 2013;170(7):768–81.
32. Lipsitz JD, Martin LY, Mannuzza S, Chapman TF, Liebowitz MR, Klein DF, et al. Childhood separation anxiety disorder in patients with adult anxiety disorders. Am J Psychiatry. 1994;151(6):927–9.
33. Gesi C, Abelli M, Cardini A, Lari L, Di Paolo L, Silove D, et al. Separation anxiety disorder from the perspective of DSM-5: clinical investigation among subjects with panic disorder and associations with mood disorders spectrum. CNS Spectr. 2016;21(1):70–5.
34. Elbay RY, Gormez A, Kilic A, Avci SH. Separation anxiety disorder among outpatients with major depressive disorder: prevalence and clinical correlates. Compr Psychiatry. 2021;105:152219.
35. Shear MK, Simon N, Wall M, Zisook S, Neimeyer R, Duan N, et al. Complicated grief and related bereavement issues for DSM-5. Depress Anxiety. 2011;28(2):103–17.
36. Silove D, Momartin S, Marnane C, Steel Z, Manicavasagar V. Adult separation anxiety disorder among war-affected Bosnian refugees: comorbidity with PTSD and associations with dimensions of trauma. J Trauma Stress. 2010;23(1):169–72.

37. Cyranowski JM, Frank E, Young E, Shear MK. Adolescent onset of the gender difference in lifetime rates of major depression: a theoretical model. Arch Gen Psychiatry. 2000;57(1):21–7.
38. Cyranowski JM, Bookwala J, Feske U, Houck P, Pilkonis P, Kostelnik B. Adult attachment profiles, interpersonal difficulties, and response to interpersonal psychotherapy in women with recurrent major depression. J Soc Clin Psychol. 2002;21(2):191–217.
39. Milrod B, Markowitz JC, Gerber AJ, Cyranowski J, Altemus M, Shapiro T, et al. Childhood separation anxiety and the pathogenesis and treatment of adult anxiety. Am J Psychiatry. 2014;171(1):34–43.
40. Verduin TL, Kendall PC. Differential occurrence of comorbidity within childhood anxiety disorders. J Clin Child Adolesc Psychol. 2003;32(2):290–5.
41. Silove D, Marnane C, Wagner R, Manicavasagar V. Associations of personality disorder with early separation anxiety in patients with adult separation anxiety disorder. J Personal Disord. 2011;25(1):128–33.
42. Kotov R, Krueger RF, Watson D, Cicero DC, Conway CC, DeYoung CG, et al. The hierarchical taxonomy of psychopathology (HiTOP): a quantitative nosology based on consensus of evidence. Annu Rev Clin Psychol. 2021;17:83–108.
43. Kotov R, Krueger RF, Watson D, Achenbach TM, Althoff RR, Bagby RM, et al. The hierarchical taxonomy of psychopathology (HiTOP): a dimensional alternative to traditional nosologies. J Abnorm Psychol. 2017;126(4):454–77.
44. Watson D, Forbes MK, Levin-Aspenson HF, Ruggero CJ, Kotelnikova Y, Khoo S, et al. The development of preliminary HiTOP internalizing spectrum scales. Assessment. 2021;29(1):17–33. https://doi.org/10.1177/10731911211003976.

Separation Anxiety and Other Anxiety Disorders

Barbara Milrod

A tension runs through the recent literature on adult separation anxiety disorder (SEPAD). Contrasting views of separation anxiety are described by the necessarily phenomenological focus required for DSM diagnosis, captured by standard diagnostic measures [1–3] that perforce require patients' relatively ready acknowledgment of symptoms and anxiety experienced with separations from one or more close attachment figures. This stands in contrast to a broader clinical appreciation of aspects of separation anxiety and its manifestations that cannot always be captured by assessment and diagnostic instruments [4]. This divergence between even the very best semi-structured assessment measures that have been developed to assess SEPAD and clinical phenomena as recognized by experienced clinicians *per se* is more noticeable in SEPAD than in any of the other anxiety disorders or PTSD [5]. The disparity occurs as a result of the well-described ego-syntonic quality of separation anxiety [5, 6], which differs markedly from the other anxiety disorders. Both ego-syntonicity and lack of appreciation of its manifestations, even among many who suffer with SEPAD makes its epidemiological measurement complicated and may contribute to its well-described cultural variance [5, 7, 8]. It is this divergence between the ego-syntonic aspects of separation anxiety and its more jarring, disruptive, and noticeable (ego-dystonic) components that in part necessarily accounts for such an uncommonly wide range of prevalence rates across cultures [6–8]. Not all cultures and ethnic groups treat anxiety experienced during separations from loved ones in the same way [7, 8].

B. Milrod (✉)
Psychiatry and Behavioral Science (PRIME), Albert Einstein College of Medicine, New York, NY, USA

Faculty of the New York Psychoanalytic Institute and the Columbia Psychoanalytic Institute for Training and Research, New York, NY, USA
e-mail: bmilrod@montefiore.org

S. Pini, B. Milrod (eds.), *Separation Anxiety in Adulthood*,
https://doi.org/10.1007/978-3-031-37446-3_5

People suffering from separation anxiety are likely to come from highly anxious families and to have mothers/primary caretakers for whom separations are anxiety-provoking and stressful [9, 10]. Yet family, parental, and cultural styles of anxiety surrounding separations can normalize the symptoms of SEPAD within these highly anxious families, making symptoms blend into what feels (and is, for most affected families) like normal life [4–6]. Some of these problems have become exaggerated since the COVID pandemic, with families who have high anxiety levels who may (or may not) have suffered losses clinging to one another with even more intensity than they did before the lockdown [11]. As in other anxiety disorders that feature high levels of avoidance, symptoms of SEPAD may be apparently minimized provided that the sufferer does not make attempts to undertake actions that provoke anxiety, such as planning to be away from their close attachment object, or to leave home. Home in SEPAD can come to signify a primary attachment relationship [12]. In the case of SEPAD, often entire family systems and cultural milieus reinforce the sense of danger and profound reluctance about separations [4]. Furthermore, the stress of parenting has also been shown to be worse for parents who have experienced significant trauma, and leads to higher incidence of childhood separation anxiety [13–15]. Thus, people suffering from SEPAD may not always immediately recognize that the anxiety they experience separating from close attachment objects is problematic, or that separation and greater independence constitutes an emotional achievement they have not yet accomplished, or may feel ambivalent about accomplishing [16]. Patients may not experience life-limiting anxiety until they are faced with their own inability to master age-expectable average developmental norms, such as going to college or trying to spend time away from home in ways that are socially expected [16]. This problem, which affects understanding of the prevalence and clinical appreciation of the wide range of manifestations of the effects of SEPAD [6, 17], including ways in which manifestations of SEPAD affect development of broader comorbid mood and anxiety disorders [6], can be reinforced by separation anxiety patients' tendency to experience their terror and sense of inadequacy physically via somatic symptoms and discomfort, in much the same way that patients with panic disorder can experience anxiety somatically [4, 6, 16]. Recognition that SEPAD symptoms have an emotional origin can itself take time [4].

1 Clinical Example

Ms. R brought her 3-year-old daughter Lucy to see a child psychiatrist when Lucy's pre-school refused to permit Lucy to continue in school without an evaluation. Two months into her 3's program, Lucy remained mute in school every day, she wept constantly every day after her mother left her, and throughout the 2 hours of her daily pre-school program, Lucy stood by the window of the classroom, gazing at the street after her mother, anxiously awaiting her return. She was unable to participate in any of the activities in school.

During the initial parent evaluation of Ms. R, mother denied suffering from any anxiety about separating from Lucy. She seemed stymied and confused that Lucy was so miserable and frightened in school. "It's a nice place," Ms. R commented. Ms. R inquired as to how the therapist's meeting with Lucy, scheduled for later that week, would transpire. "She may not leave me," Ms. R said. "We'll have to see." The therapist assured Ms. R that she would do her best.

When the therapist first met Lucy, Ms. R walked her to the door of the office, bent over Lucy, and stood rigidly in a manner that both hovered over Lucy's small form and also blocked Lucy's access to entering the office. Ms. R's nonverbal communication indicated physically that she anticipated that Lucy would find it frightening to meet the therapist or enter her office without her, and that she, Ms. R, was positioned to provide protection. When the therapist reached around the mother's form to shake Lucy's hand in greeting, Lucy entered the office without her mother. Ms. R seemed surprised, and the therapist told Ms. R that she could wait in the waiting room, a few steps from the office door.

During her next meeting with Ms. R, the therapist said that it had seemed as though Ms. R was anxious or uncomfortable separating from Lucy at the door to her office (Lucy, having been given the small nonverbal encouragement from the therapist, had done well with this separation). Ms. R was genuinely shocked to hear this. "I believe that you are more anxious about separating from Lucy than you had been aware," the therapist told the mother. With encouragement, mother sought her own psychiatric help for her own separation anxiety, which, in addition to Lucy's own therapy, helped to curb Lucy's severe and crippling symptoms and permitted her to function normally in pre-school within the month.

From a purely phenomenologic perspective, patients with SEPAD feel highly anxious when they are physically separated from close, needed attachment figures. Anxiety can equally arise when anything that might threaten (even in fantasy) the proximity or availability of this attachment relationship, such as during anticipated age-normative developmental experiences of gradually increasing autonomy, like going on sleepover dates, trips away from home, or going to college [4]. These age-normative expectable developmental separations become points of recognition of psychopathology in patients with SEPAD at times when the requirement for mother or other close attachment figures are no longer normative [6]. As illustrated in the case example above, separation anxiety can also commonly occur among parents when they are expected to be apart from their children.

Panic disorder, agoraphobia, and SEPAD. The longitudinal developmental progression from SEPAD to gradual development of agoraphobia and panic disorder [7, 18] has been well documented. The dominance of the link/progression from SEPAD to panic and agoraphobia has been argued to arise in part out of the DSM III's formulation of panic disorder's dominance as a model of endogenous anxiety among anxiety disorders [7]. Even so, carefully conducted, large scale epidemiological studies and a comprehensive meta-analysis of case control, prospective, and retrospective studies [8, 17, 19] have demonstrated the link between childhood separation anxiety disorder and later development of panic disorder and other anxiety disorders [17, 19]. Symptoms of agoraphobia, wherein patients can experience extreme discomfort and panic-level disorganizing anxiety when they leave their home or narrow neighborhood or other familiar, magically-designated "safe spaces"

[4, 20] can gradually arise out of symptoms of earlier SEPAD, in situations in which the home comes to symbolically represent the primary attachment relationship, such as with mother [12].

Viewing these common symptomatic progressions through a psychodynamic lens can be informative, because it permits acknowledgment and incorporation of the human mind's universal use of symbolic logic [21–23]. The underlying emotional pressures of SEPAD and those of agoraphobia, particularly when the patient feels the need for a phobic companion, are densely intertwined [24]. From a SEPAD perspective, the phobic companion is almost always the person, often the mother or her representative, from whom separation feels terrifying and intolerable in the dyadic anxiety-relationship that forms the core matrix of both perceived safety: fragile and dependent on the presence of an external attachment relationship as it is, and the danger of separation anxiety and being apart from this person. Therapeutic relationships with physicians of any specialty when treatment is regular, or with psychopharmacologists or psychotherapists of any orientation can mirror core aspects of this complicated ambivalent yet controlling attachment, re-enacted in the universal phenomenon of transference [24–26]. Helena Deutsch [24] in her groundbreaking paper "The genesis of agoraphobia" articulated both the dense, controlling, yet also passive underpinnings to the attachment to the phobic companion in agoraphobia, which encompasses often disorganizing and disavowed rage. One of the underlying terrors is that the person feels unable to function on their own, aggravating rage and anxiety. These same organizing dynamisms of disavowed, usually only partially conscious rage are also prominent in SEPAD [27].

Parental, mostly maternal, diagnosis of major depression, panic disorder, and particularly separation anxiety disorder *per se* have been connected to development of childhood SEPAD [17, 18, 28]. Yet this is not universally true; it appears that core elements of family style and epigenetic factors as well as maternal trauma have important roles to play in development of separation anxiety [6, 29, 30]. Clinically, a crucial element in development of SEPAD seems to be parents' inability to tolerate their child's anxiety and/or discomfort, no matter what the parent's diagnosis [16, 31]. On the ground, the terrified child, who, for example, is frightened of sleeping alone in their bed, encounters parent(s) who neither can soothe them nor can effectively tolerate or set limits with the childhood terror of separation anxiety as enacted in the fundamental separation paradigm of sleeping in one's own bed [6]. Escalating rage and anxiety can follow in both parent(s) and children, with separation (in this example, for everyone to go to sleep at night) burdened with catastrophic fantasies of loss, rage, rage-filled fantasies, and terror [16, 32].

It is in this way that early, formative, in this case insecure, dysregulated childhood attachment relationships cast a long shadow on later development of insecure, dysregulated adult attachment relationships [33], with broad manifestations across the ability to develop more stable relationship patterns with others [6, 33–35]. These underlying formative attachment relationships and dynamisms have a direct effect on the relative lack of ease with which such patients are able to seek social support under traumatic circumstances [36, 37]. Lack of social supports has a direct influence on vulnerability to the development of PTSD with exposure to trauma, for example. People with longstanding or underlying separation anxiety have higher rates of developing PTSD with trauma [36]. This link is likely mediated by the SEPAD sufferer's higher resting state of anxiety, as well as their inability to obtain adequate social support [38, 39]. Presence of separation anxiety affects the—crucial—general ability to self-soothe, which is also a key to maintaining a sense of stability under uncertain or stressful circumstances [6, 34, 35, 40]. The central abilities to modulate and tolerate blasts of affect are similarly affected [33–37, 40].

References

1. Cyranowski JM, Shear MK, Rucci P, Fagiolini A, Frank E, Grochocinski VJ, Cassano G. Adult separation anxiety: psychometric properties of a new structured clinical interview. J Psychiatr Res. 2002;36:77–86.
2. Manicavasagar V, Silove D, Wagner R, Drobny J. A self-report questionnaire for measuring separation anxiety in adulthood. Compr Psychiatry. 2003;44:146–53.
3. Silove D, Manicavasagar V, O'Connell D, Blaszczynski A, Wagner R, Henry J. The development of the separation anxiety symptom inventory (SASI). Aust N Z J Psychiatry. 1993;27:477–88.
4. Busch F, Milrod B, Singer M, Aronson A. Panic focused psychodynamic psychotherapy: eXtended range: psychodynamic psychotherapy for anxiety disorders: a transdiagnostic treatment manual. Taylor & Francis, LLC: Milton Park; 2012.
5. Milrod B. An epidemiological contribution to clinical understanding of anxiety. Am J Psychiatr. 2015;172:601–2.
6. Milrod B, Markowitz JC, Gerber AJ, Cyranowski J, Altemus M, Shapiro T, Hofer M, Glatt C. Childhood separation anxiety and the pathogenesis and treatment of adult anxiety. Am J Psychiatr. 2014;171:34–43.
7. Manicavasagar V, Silove D. Separation anxiety in adults, clinical features, diagnostic dilemmas and treatment guidelines. London: Elsevier, Academic Press; 2020.
8. Silove D, Alonso J, Bromet E, et al. Pediatric-onset and adult-onset separation anxiety disorder across countries in the World Mental Health Survey. Am J Psychiatry. 2015;172:647–56.
9. Last CG, Hersen M, Kazdin AE, Francis G, Grubb HJ. Psychiatric illness in the mothers of anxious children. Am J Psychiatry. 1987;144(12):1580–3.
10. Orgilés M, Penosa P, Morales A, Fernández-Martínez I, Espada JP. Maternal anxiety and separation anxiety in children aged between 3 and 6 years: the mediating role of parenting style. J Dev Behav Pediatr. 2018;39(8):621–8.
11. Markowitz JC. In the aftermath of the pandemic: interpersonal psychotherapy for anxiety, depression, and PTSD. New York: OUP; 2021.
12. Milrod B. Unconscious pregnancy fantasies in patients with panic disorder. J Am Psychoanal Assoc. 1998;46:673–90.
13. Chemtob CM, Nomura Y, Rajendran K, Yehuda R, Schwartz D, Abramovitz R. Impact of maternal posttraumatic stress disorder and depression following exposure to the September 11 attacks on preschool children's behavior: impact of PTSD and depression. Child Dev. 2010;81:1129–41. https://doi.org/10.1111/j.1467-8624.2010.01458.x.
14. Cho B, Woods-Jaeger B, Borelli J. Parenting stress moderates the relation between parental trauma exposure and child anxiety symptoms. Child Psychiatry Hum Dev. 2021;52:1050–9. https://doi.org/10.1007/s10578-020-01087-1.
15. Fonagy P, Gergely G, Jurist E, Target M. Afect regulation, mentalization, and the development of the self. Other Press; 2002.
16. Preter S, Shapiro T, Milrod B. Child and adolescent anxiety psychodynamic psychotherapy: a manual. Oxford: Oxford University Press; 2018. Print ISBN-13:9780190877712.

17. Kossowsky J, Pfaltz MC, Schneider S, Taeymans J, Locher C, Gaab J. The separation anxiety hypothesis of panic disorder revisited: a meta-analysis. Am J Psychiatry. 2013;170(7):768–81. https://doi.org/10.1176/appi.ajp.2012.12070893.
18. Biederman J, Petty CR, Hirshfeld-Becker DR, Henin A, Faraone SV, Fraire M, Henry B, McQuade J, Rosenbaum JF. Developmental trajectories of anxiety disorders in offspring at high risk for panic disorder and major depression. Psychiatry Res. 2007;153(3):245–52.
19. Roberson-Nay R, Eaves RJ, Hettema JM, Kendler KS, Silberg JL. Childhood separation anxiety disorder and adult onset panic attacks share a common genetic diathesis. Depress Anxiety. 2012;29:320–7.
20. Milrod B. Emptiness in agoraphobia. J Am Psychoanal Assoc. 2007;55:1007–26.
21. Freud S. The interpretation of dreams. In: The complete works of Sigmund Freud, SE, vol. 4. Hogarth Press London; 1900.
22. Roose SP, Glick RA. Anxiety as symptom and signal. Hillsdale, NJ: The Analytic Press; 1995.
23. Wentura D. Cognition and emotion: on paradigms and metaphors. Cogn Emot. 2019;33(1):85–93. https://doi.org/10.1080/02699931.2019.1567464.
24. Deutsch H. The genesis of agoraphobia. Int J Psychoanal. 1929;10:51–69.
25. Freud S. Fragment of an analysis of a case of hysteria. S.E. V 1905;7:3–124.
26. Milrod B, Cooper A, Shear MK. Psychodynamic concepts of anxiety. In: Stein DJ, Hollander E, editors. Chapter in textbook of anxiety disorders. Washington, DC: American Psychiatric Press; 2001. p. 89–103.
27. Busch F, Milrod B. Psychodynamic treatment for separation anxiety in a treatment nonresponder. JAPA. 2015;63:893–919.
28. Cooper PJ, Fearn V, Willetts L, Seabrook H, Parkinson M. Affective disorder in the parents of a clinic sample of children with anxiety disorders. J Affect Disord. 2006;93(1–3):205–12.
29. Hirshfeld DR, Biederman J, Brody L, Faraone SV, Rosenbaum JF. Associations between expressed emotion and child behavioral inhibition and psychopathology: a pilot study. J Am Acad Child Adolesc Psychiatry. 1997;36(2):205–13.
30. Schwerdtfeger KL, Goff BSN. Intergenerational transmission of trauma: exploring mother–infant prenatal attachment. J Trauma Stress. 2007;20:39–51. https://doi.org/10.1002/jts.20179.
31. Milrod B. A 9 year-old with conversion disorder, successfully treated with psychoanalysis. Int J Psychoanal. 2002;83:623–31.
32. Milrod B, Busch F, Cooper A, Shapiro T. Manual of panic - focused psychodynamic psychotherapy. Washington, DC: APA Press; 1997.
33. Fonagy P, Target M, Gergely G. Attachment and borderline personality disorder. A theory and some evidence. Psychiatr Clin North Am. 2000;23(1):103–22.
34. Bowlby J. Attachment and loss. New York: Basic Books; 1973.
35. Bowlby J. A secure base: parent-child attachment and healthy human development. London: Routledge; 1988. p. 5.
36. Markowitz JC, Milrod B, Bleiberg KL, Marshall RD. Interpersonal factors in understanding and treating posttraumatic stress disorder. J Psychiatr Pract. 2009;15:133–40.
37. Markowitz JC, Lipsitz J, Milrod BL. A critical review of outcome research on interpersonal psychotherapy for anxiety disorders. Depress Anxiety. 2014;31(4):316–25.
38. Bleiberg KL, Markowitz JC. Interpersonal psychotherapy for posttraumatic stress disorder. Am J Psychiatry. 2005;162:181–3.
39. Krupnick JL, Green BL, Stockton P, et al. Group interpersonal psychotherapy with low-income women with posttraumatic stress disorder. Psychother Res. 2008;18:497–507.
40. Busch F, Milrod B, Chen C, Singer M. Trauma-focused psychodynamic psychotherapy. Bringing evidence-based psychodynamic treatment to patients with PTSD. Oxford: Oxford University Press; 2021.

Separation Anxiety and Posttraumatic Stress Disorder

John C. Markowitz and Barbara Milrod

Separation anxiety disorder (SAD) and posttraumatic stress disorder (PTSD) share numerous clinical features, which may be no accident. Information on their relationship is limited partly because separation anxiety has only recently been recognized as a problem affecting adults. Nonetheless, the two disorders appear to overlap in high chronicity, long delay to treatment, high comorbidity with one another, significant social and functional impairment, as well as a possible relationship in treatment response (Table 1). Moreover, individuals with each disorder share aspects of a clinical presentation involving affect dysregulation and mistrust of the safety of their environment. Because both tend to be chronic disorders, often arising in childhood, disentangling the two can be difficult. Nonetheless, this chapter explores the relationship between the two.

J. C. Markowitz (✉)
Columbia University Vagelos College of Physicians and Surgeons, New York, NY, USA

New York State Psychiatric Institute, New York, NY, USA
e-mail: Jcm42@cumc.columbia.edu

B. Milrod
Psychiatry and Behavioral Science (PRIME), Albert Einstein College of Medicine, New York, NY, USA
e-mail: bmilrod@montefiore.org

S. Pini, B. Milrod (eds.), *Separation Anxiety in Adulthood*,
https://doi.org/10.1007/978-3-031-37446-3_6

Table 1 Comparison of Separation Anxiety Disorder and PTSD

	Separation anxiety disorder	Posttraumatic stress disorder
Lifetime prevalence	4.8%	6.8%
Predominant affect	Anxiety	Anxiety
Chronicity	High	High
Mean delay to treatment (years)	23	12
Response to affect-focused therapy?	Possibly	Yes

1 Separation Anxiety Disorder

The DSM-5 defines Separation Anxiety Disorder (F93.0) as "excessive or unwarranted fear or anxiety due to separation from whoever he or she is attached to," as demonstrated by at least three of eight anxious symptoms [1]. The individual feels helpless, unsafe, and anxious away from the presence of a significant other. That is, the environment feels unsafe absent the other. From a stress-diathesis perspective, SAD reflects some combination of temperament, genetic or epigenetic vulnerability and environmental insult, such as highly anxious parenting [2]. Although SAD often arises in early childhood, adult onset does occur. In a multinational World Health Organization survey of nearly 39,000 individuals, Silove and colleagues found a lifetime SAD prevalence of 4.8% and 1-year prevalence of approximately 1.0% [3]. Despite the clinical assumption that SAD begins early in life, 43.8% of reported lifetime cases reported onset after age 18 [3]. SAD is chronic, in part because individuals and their families consider such behavior unremarkable and ego-syntonic, and hence seek no treatment [2, 4]. One study found SAD was the diagnosis with longest mean delay to treatment, approaching an average of 23 years [5]. (By contrast, the mean time to treatment for bipolar disorder was 6 years.)

2 Posttraumatic Stress Disorder

Over the course of a lifetime, most people suffer exposure to a traumatic event severe enough to qualify for Criterion A of the DSM PTSD diagnosis [1]. As most people are resilient, only a subset – 6.8% -- develops the disorder post trauma [6]. Individuals who develop PTSD have an anxious, shattered, mistrustful sense of the dangers of their environment, including the people in it [7]. They withdraw from social supports, even though social supports protect against PTSD [8, 9]. Like SAD, PTSD may begin early in life (for example, consequent to child abuse) or have later onset. People at high risk of trauma (for example, military personnel) face greater risk of developing PTSD, and those with a traumatic event history (DSM-5 Criterion A) often suffer "revictimization," experiencing multiple, reinforcing traumas [10]. Finding their emotions overwhelming, people with PTSD struggle to suppress them, often reporting feeling nothing, numb to emotion (DSM-5 PTSD Criterion D.6) [1]; yet the underlying affect tends to be anxiety. Individuals with PTSD, too, have a long latency to seeking treatment, an average of 12 years [5].

Although the DSM-5 definition of PTSD emphasizes cognitive and behavioral symptoms, the disorder has strong interpersonal elements [7]. Both PTSD and SAD can be considered disorders of dysregulated attachment. As other sections of this book elaborate at length, separation anxiety in effect epitomizes insecure attachment: the individual feels uncomfortable without the immediate presence of a protective other [11]. In PTSD, too, emotions are dysregulated. Having experienced overwhelming events, individuals with PTSD respond with overwhelming negative affects – horror, fear, anger, sadness, rage – that they find unbearable and attempt to suppress. Many become affectively distanced, depersonalized, and numb in a futile attempt to suppress these emotions. The emotions then tend to surface spasmodically, unexpectedly, and uncontrollably – a man in a pharmacy explodes at the person shuffling ahead of him in line – reinforcing the sense that feelings are dangerous and require suppression [7].

Suppressing affect has considerable interpersonal cost. People with PTSD, having been traumatized by external events, understandably mistrust their environment and the people in it. Lack of trust is a key interpersonal element of the syndrome. Yet because they have suppressed their feelings, they are unable to read the environment, which frequently leads to mistrust of trustworthy people and revictimization by untrustworthy others [7].

3 Commonalities and Differences

Silove and colleagues found that antecedent SAD was a risk factor for PTSD (odds ratio = 1.6) [3]. In clinical samples, SAD has been found to be a risk factor for PTSD in children who have suffered burns [12] or missile attacks [13]. In our treatment sample of 29 military veterans with chronic PTSD, 69% had comorbid SAD [14]. Perhaps surprisingly, Silove et al. did not find the reverse relationship between the disorders: i.e., PTSD did not predict subsequent development of SAD (OR = 0.9) [3]. Yet as we have noted [14], a reciprocal relationship may in fact exist. In that large WHO study, risk factors for SAD included childhood adversity, "maladaptive family functioning," and extreme childhood traumas [3] that can produce early childhood symptoms resembling PTSD [15].

Thus, SAD and PTSD each involve interpersonal insecurity, insecure attachment, emotional dysregulation, and they may be highly comorbid. The presence of SAD constitutes a risk factor for PTSD, and if the reverse has not been demonstrated, it seems that the two syndromes share common underlying features. At the same time, these fellow travelers notably differ in some respects. Insecure attachment has different features and different expression. In SAD, anxiety is more freely communicated in the context of threatened or actual separation, whereas in PTSD, insecure attachment often presents as detachment: emotions are suppressed as dangerous, hence not easily accessible.

What predisposes some individuals to develop PTSD, when most of those exposed to trauma do not? As PTSD is a complex and heterogeneous disorder, no single answer suffices. Severity and chronicity of traumas surely matter. One important factor, however, appears to be attachment-related and can be at least partially conceptualized as involving separation anxiety. As Silove and colleagues noted, a meta-analysis of community studies [16] suggests that SAD "may represent a generic risk factor for a range of anxiety disorders and other psychopathology in adulthood," [3, p. 648] although that meta-analysis did not address the overlap of SAD with PTSD. We have postulated that separation anxiety arising from early family environment dysfunction and trauma may mediate onset of disorders including PTSD [2, 7, 17].

Childhood trauma seems likely to engender both disorders. Childhood abuse or trauma can yield insecure attachment [18, 19], including its manifestation as separation anxiety. Childhood abuse and trauma can also cause or induce later vulnerability to PTSD. An individual with insecure attachment is less likely to feel comfortable in interpersonal encounters, hence likely to have both fewer confidants and less trust in confiding in them [7, 17]. Should that individual encounter a trauma, he or she is less likely than a securely attached individual to reach out to others for social support. Research indicates that such social support and emotional processing of trauma protects against developing PTSD [8, 9]. An insecurely attached individual, already less trustful of others and with fewer supports to turn to, may well keep the trauma and its associated feelings internalized, increasing the risk of developing PTSD [7–9, 17, 20].

This interpersonal, attachment- and affect-based perspective provides an alternative to the cognitive- behavioral fight/flight theory that has long dominated PTSD research [7, 21].

4 Treatment Findings

In our research using interpersonal psychotherapy (IPT), an affect-focused psychotherapy, to treat PTSD, we have long sought to explore dysregulated attachment as a potential moderating or mediating factor in the interpersonal treatment of PTSD [17]. Although unable to accurately assess it in our initial randomized controlled study [21], we subsequently did so in an open 14-week IPT trial for 29 military veterans with chronic PTSD [14]. In that study, in addition to measuring PTSD and depressive symptoms, we assessed two aspects of dysregulated attachment: Symptom-Specific Reflective Function (SSRF) [22], a measure of one aspect of mentalization, or Reflective Function [23], that assesses patients' emotional understanding of their PTSD symptoms; and the Structured Clinical Interview for Separation Anxiety Symptoms (SCI-SAS) [24], which assesses childhood and adult separation anxiety.

The study, funded by the American Psychoanalytic Association Fund for Psychoanalytic Research, had two goals. The first was to assess the prevalence of SAD in this patient sample of veterans with chronic PTSD. No research had previously evaluated SAD in PTSD. Second, we explored the clinical associations of SAD and PTSD, including both the effect of having SAD on PTSD outcome, and the effect of a brief interpersonal PTSD (IPT for PTSD) treatment on adult SAD symptoms. Among our hypotheses were that (1) SAD prevalence in this PTSD sample would be high; that (2) initially low mentalization and dysregulated attachment (measured by SSRF) and (3) adult separation anxiety symptoms (measured by SCI-SAS) would improve with acute IPT treatment; and (4) early change in mentalization between baseline and week 4 would predict PTSD outcome at week 14 [14]. No prior research had explored the relationships between SAD and PTSD in a treatment context.

5 Methods

The study employed the best available assessment measures, administered by trained and reliable interviewers and raters. PTSD and depressive symptoms were assessed using the Clinician-Administered PTSD Scale (CAPS-5 [25]) and 17-item Hamilton Depression Rating Scale (Ham-D [26]), respectively, at weeks 0, 7, and 14. The RF/SSRF interview was conducted at weeks 0, 4, and 14, as was the SCI-SAS. Because SSRF, here adapted to address patients' emotional understanding of their PTSD symptoms, seems more sensitive to acute change than general RF, which reflects mentalization of core relationships, we focused on the former in this brief trial. SSRF scores range from −1 to 9, with a score of 5 being normative [22].

The SCI-SAS is a 16-item scale equally divided between childhood and adult separation anxiety items. Each item is scored between 0 and 2; a score of 8 or more defines clinically significant, syndromal SAD [24]. The SCI-SAS has excellent psychometric properties. Because childhood items are assessed retrospectively, only adult SAD is expected to change with intervention. To assess separation anxiety change, severity was assessed by summing the total score [24].

Relatively inexperienced therapists, postdoctoral or newly minted psychologists, delivered 14 weekly sessions of interpersonal psychotherapy (IPT) for PTSD under the first author's supervision. This therapy does not employ exposure to trauma reminders, as cognitive behavioral therapies for PTSD do. Instead, IPT focuses on patients' emotions and their utility in negotiating interpersonal relationships and re-establishing trust [7, 21]. This involves initial affective attunement to penetrate numbness, helping patients to identify and validate their emotions and to see negative affects as interpersonally informative. Once in touch with their emotions, patients used them to strengthen social supports and to determine who is trustworthy and who is not. For example, anger generally means someone feels mistreated. If a patient felt angry about an interpersonal encounter, he or she might role-play confronting the other person. If the other responded with an acknowledgment or apology, he or she might be trustworthy. If not, then recognition that the other person is untrustworthy, upsetting as that might be, has been learned. This non-exposure, affect-focused IPT approach worked as well as the best tested exposure therapy in a randomized controlled trial [21].

6 Results

The 29 veterans had a mean age of 43.3 (SD = 14.1). Nine (31%) were women; 31% described themselves as African American and 14% as Hispanic. Of the 29 veterans with CAPS-5-diagnosed chronic PTSD assessed for SAD by SCI-SAS, 69% also met SAD criteria. Separation anxiety did not correlate with baseline PTSD severity, depressive severity, or age when traumatized. Patients with and without comorbid SAD had comparable PTSD and depression severity.

Both PTSD and depressive symptoms responded to IPT. Twenty-two patients, including 17 with comorbid SAD, completed the 14-week course of IPT. Those 17 with baseline comorbid SAD reported significantly improved adult separation anxiety ($p = 0.009$). Adult SAD improvements predicted improvement in depression ($p = 0.049$). Patients with SAD had a stronger relationship between early SSRF gains and subsequent adult SAD improvement ($p = 0.021$) than patients without SAD. Of the 17 patients with baseline SAD who had week 14 SCI-SAS scores, 6 (35%) no longer met criteria for significant SAD and six (35%) reported an at least 50% decrement in adult SCI-SAS score, indicating treatment response. Five patients (29%) met both criteria for improvement. Of nine completers with DSM-5-defined SAD, five patients fell under diagnostic threshold post treatment ("remission," 56%).

This study was the first of its kind. As a small, pilot open trial, its findings are preliminary and require replication. Nonetheless, the results are exciting and make intuitive clinical sense. The prevalence of separation anxiety disorder among veterans with chronic PTSD was quite high, comparable to the 80% Milrod et al. reported in a patient sample with patients with anxiety disorders who had not responded to prior evidence-based treatment [27]. Patients with dysregulated attachment improved on multiple measures over the course of just 14 weekly sessions of IPT, a non-exposure, affect- and relationship-focused treatment for PTSD. Although IPT targeted PTSD and depression rather than SAD, SAD also acutely improved. This is a novel finding given the dearth of systematic outcomes studies on treatment of SAD. More broadly, the results hint at the potential attachment-related mechanism of an affect-focused therapy in both relieving PTSD and depressive symptoms and in repairing dysregulated attachment.

7 PTSD/SAD Case

Mr. A., a 42-year-old married father of two, described worsening PTSD symptoms since the death of his father several years before. Abused throughout childhood, he reported frequent nightmares of "losing everything" and sudden, vicious panic attacks. He startled easily. He alternated between feeling numb and pointless and extreme irritability and anxiety. When irritable, he said hostile and provocative things to his wife, his most frequent target, ultimately provoking her to consider divorce. The idea that she might leave filled Mr. A with terror, as he was profoundly sensitive and anxious when she left the house even to go to work. He lived in a liminal state, torn between being "sick" of her and terror of losing her. Small interpersonal distances from her felt enormous.

Throughout childhood, Mr. A had witnessed his father physically abusing three successive wives and several step-siblings. His father beat them with belts and wires, often screaming insults at them and everyone else. While not beaten himself, Mr. A always worried he would be next. He felt a "hopeless, pathetic" urge, particularly as a small child, to protect his family members. His mother had made a near-lethal suicide attempt when he was 4 years old after a beating by his monstrous, larger than life father. Mr. A could recall "howling in pain" at the time, and in reconstructing the events of his childhood, said that he never felt safe.

His father constantly verbally attacked him about his inadequacy as a man. Relentlessly, into Mr. A's 20s, his father asserted that he could never hope to amount to anything. Mr. A quietly agreed: he considered himself inadequate in all respects. Like his father, he considered any display of emotion childish, unmanly, weak, and "histrionic," a favorite paternal insult. Feeling consistently disgusted with himself, Mr. A stayed close to his mother, almost never leaving her sight before her death when he was 17. After she died, he began a series of serially monogamous relationships with women featuring the same ambivalence, severe separation problems, chronic dissatisfaction, and detachment punctuated with explosive outbursts that characterized his current relationship with his wife.

A 14-week course of IPT focused not on this foundational history but on Mr. A's feelings in current relationships, addressing in the present the important links between his emotions and relational patterns. Early sessions focused on affective attunement [7], helping the patient to recognize how he felt in particular daily encounters and to understand that feelings were informative rather than a weakness. In particular, he recognized that his anger need not be a dangerous, "bad" emotion like his father's but a signal and opportunity to tell his wife when she was bothering him. With role play to modulate his delivery of this message, and with her cooperation, his tentative trust in their relationship grew and the marital situation improved. His PTSD and adult separation anxiety symptoms decreased significantly.

8 Summary

The relationship between separation anxiety and posttraumatic stress disorder is not entirely clear because the research connecting them has been so limited. Nonetheless, the two disorders appear intimately connected and to share roots in dysregulated attachment [11, 14]. We speculate that affect-focused therapies such as IPT and psychodynamic psychotherapy may share a treatment path and even neurobiological connections [28] through addressing attachment issues in PTSD, anxiety disorders such as panic disorder, and separation anxiety disorder [11, 27]. How comfortable you feel with others and how you handle your emotions matters. It is exciting to consider that affect-focused brief therapies may work through repairing dysregulated attachment to increase interpersonal stability and the ability to mobilize protective social supports. More work needs to be done to elucidate these connections.

References

1. American Psychiatric Association. Diagnostic and statistical manual of mental disorders, Fifth Edition (DSM-5). Arlington, VA: American Psychiatric Association; 2013.
2. Milrod B, Markowitz JC, Gerber AJ, Cyranowski J, Altemus M, Shapiro T, Hofer M, Glatt C. Childhood separation anxiety and the pathogenesis and treatment of adult anxiety. Am J Psychiatry. 2014;171:34–43.

3. Silove D, Alonso J, Bromet E, Gruber M, Sampson N, Scott K, Andrade L, Benjet C, Caldas de Almeida JM, De Girolamo G, de Jonge P, Demyttenaere K, Fiestas F, Florescu S, Gureje O, He Y, Karam E, Lepine JP, Murphy S, Villa-Posada J, Zarkov Z, Kessler RC. Pediatric-onset and adult-onset separation anxiety disorder across countries in the World Mental Health Survey. Am J Psychiatry. 2015;172:647–56.
4. Milrod B. An epidemiological contribution to clinical understanding of anxiety. Am J Psychiatry. 2014;172:601–2.
5. Wang PS, Berglund P, Olfson M, Pincus HA, Wells KB, Kessler RC. Failure and delay in initial treatment contact after first onset of mental disorders in the National Comorbidity Survey Replication. Arch Gen Psychiatry. 2005;62:603–13.
6. Kessler RC, Berglund P, Demler O, et al. Lifetime prevalence and age-of-onset distributions of DSM-IV disorders in the National Comorbidity Survey Replication. Arch Gen Psychiatry. 2005;62:593–602.
7. Markowitz JC. Interpersonal psychotherapy for posttraumatic stress disorder. New York: Oxford University Press; 2016.
8. Brewin CR, Andrews B, Valentine JD. Meta-analysis of risk factors for posttraumatic stress disorder in trauma-exposed adults. J Consult Clin Psychol. 2000;68:748–66.
9. Ozer EJ, Best SR, Lipsey TL, Weiss DS. Predictors of posttraumatic stress disorder and symptoms in adults: a meta-analysis. Psychol Bull. 2003;129:52–73.
10. Cloitre M, Scarvalone P, Difede JA. Posttraumatic stress disorder, self- and interpersonal dysfunction among sexually retraumatized women. J Traumatic Stress. 1997;10:437–52.
11. Diamond D. Separation anxiety and attachment dysregulation. Discussion at the American Psychoanalytic Association Scientific Paper Prize; American Psychoanalytic Annual Meeting Boston, MA June, 2021.
12. Laor N, Wolmer L, Mayes LC, Golomb A, Silverberg DS, Weizman R, Cohen DJ. Israeli preschoolers under Scud missile attacks: a developmental perspective on risk-modifying factors. Arch Gen Psychiatry. 1996;53:416–23.
13. Saxe GN, Stoddard F, Hall E, Chawla N, Lopez C, Sheridan R, King D, King L, Yehuda R. Pathways to PTSD, part I: children with burns. Am J Psychiatry. 2005;162:1299–304.
14. Milrod B, Keefe JR, Choo T-H, Arnon S, Such S, Lowell A, Neria Y, Markowitz JC. Separation anxiety in PTSD: a pilot prevalence and treatment study. Depress Anxiety. 2020;37:386–95.
15. Lieberman AF. Traumatic stress and quality of attachment: reality and internalization in disorders of infant mental health. Infant Ment Health J. 2004;25:336–51.
16. Kossowsky J, Pfaltz MC, Schneider S, Taeymans J, Locher C, Gaab J. The separation anxiety hypothesis of panic disorder revisited: a meta-analysis. Am J Psychiatry. 2013;170:768–81.
17. Markowitz JC, Milrod B, Bleiberg KL, Marshall RD. Interpersonal factors in understanding and treating posttraumatic stress disorder. J Psychiatr Pract. 2009;15:133–40.
18. Bowlby J. A secure base: parent-child attachment and healthy human development. London: Routledge; 1988.
19. Bowlby J. Attachment and loss. New York: Basic Books; 1973.
20. Guay S, Billette V, Marchand A. Exploring the links between posttraumatic stress disorder and social support: processes and potential research avenues. J Trauma Stress. 2006;19:327–38.
21. Markowitz JC, Petkova E, Neria Y, Van Meter P, Zhao Y, Hembree E, Lovell K, Biyanova T, Marshall RD. Is exposure necessary? A randomized clinical trial of interpersonal psychotherapy for PTSD. Am J Psychiatr. 2015;172:430–40.
22. Rudden MG, Milrod B, Meehan KB, Falkenstrom F. Symptom-specific reflective functioning: incorporating psychoanalytic measures into clinical trials. J Am Psychoanal Assoc. 2009;57:1473–8.
23. Fonagy P, Target M. Attachment and reflective function: their role in self-organization. Dev Psychopathol. 1997;9:679–700.
24. Cyranowski JM, Shear MK, Rucci P, Fagiolini A, Frank E, Grochocinski VJ, Kupfer DJ, Banti S, Armani A, Cassano G. Adult separation anxiety: psychometric properties of a new structured clinical interview. J Psychiatr Res. 2002;36:77–86.

25. Weathers FW, Blake DD, Schnurr PP, Kaloupek DG, Marx BP, Keane TM. The Clinician-Administered PTSD Scale for DSM-5 (CAPS-5). Interview available from the National Center for PTSD, 2013. Retrieved from www.ptsd.va.gov
26. Hamilton M. A rating scale for depression. J Neurol Neurosurg Psychiatry. 1960;23:56–62.
27. Milrod B, Altemus M, Gross C, Busch F, Silver G, Christos P, Stieber J, Schneier F. Adult separation anxiety in treatment nonresponders with anxiety disorders: delineation of the syndrome and exploration of attachment-based psychotherapy and biomarkers. Compr Psychiatry. 2016;66:139–45.
28. Suarez-Jimenez B, Zhu X, Lazarov A, Mann JJ, Schneier F, Gerber A, Barber JP, Chambless DL, Neria Y, Milrod B, Markowitz JC. Anterior hippocampal volume predicts affect-focused psychotherapy outcome. Psychol Med. 2020;50:396–402.

The Relationship Between Separation Anxiety and Bipolar Disorder

Stefano Pini, Accursio Raia, and Marianna Abelli

1 Separation Anxiety as a Potential Prodrome of Bipolar Disorder

Before detailing the relationship and reciprocal pathological effects of co-occurring separation anxiety and bipolar spectrum disorders in adulthood, we must highlight the role of childhood separation anxiety as a precursor of bipolar disorder. In 2011, the International Society for Bipolar Disorders convened a "*Taskforce on Prodromes of Bipolar Disorder*" to review scientific evidence, summarize findings on early psychopathology preceding syndromal bipolar disorder, and make research recommendations. In this process, Faedda et al. [1, 2] reviewed the research literature on prodromal features of bipolar disorder either of an affective or non-affective nature. Figure 1 is adapted from that of Faedda et al. [2]. It schematizes reviewed data that may help to characterize the pre-syndromal or prodromal phase of bipolar disorder. The potential role of separation anxiety has been added to the origin Figure based on the existing literature.

The study by Brückl et al. [3] is noteworthy within this framework. They reported and commented on Faedda et al. article as a most crucial contribution to supporting the link between separation anxiety and bipolarity. German researchers [3] found a specific association between separation anxiety in childhood with later in life (adolescence and early adulthood) bipolar disorders. Individuals with threshold SAD (all diagnostic criteria fulfilled) had an elevated risk of subsequent bipolar type I

S. Pini (✉)
Department of Clinical and Experimental Medicine, University of Pisa, Pisa, Italy
e-mail: stefano.pini@unipi.it

A. Raia · M. Abelli
Department of Clinical and Experimental Medicine, Program of Innovations in Psychiatric Treatments, School of Medicine, University of Pisa, Pisa, Italy

S. Pini, B. Milrod (eds.), *Separation Anxiety in Adulthood*,
https://doi.org/10.1007/978-3-031-37446-3_7

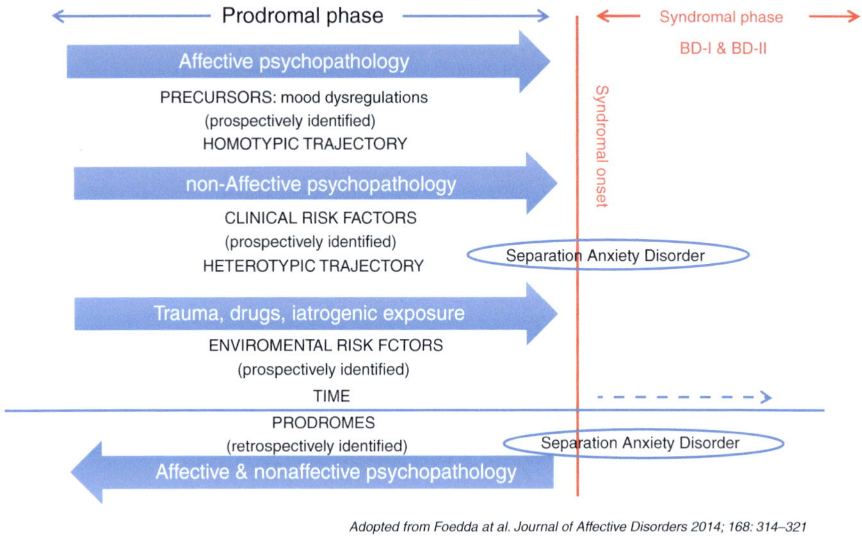

Fig. 1 Predictors of bipolar disorder

(HR = 6.2, 95% CI = 1.7–21.6) and bipolar type II disorder (HR = 8.5, 95% CI = 1.6–43.5) but not of significant depression (HR = 2.1, 95% CI = 0.7–6.0). Subthreshold (one less than full diagnostic criteria for SAD) SAD predicted the onset of bipolar disorder type II (HR = 8.1, 95% CI = 2.3–27.4) but not of bipolar disorder type I (HR = 0.6; 95% CI = 0.0–4.0) or major depression (HR = 1.5, 95% CI = 0.9–2.5). In prospectively observed cases, subthreshold or syndromal separation anxiety predicted the first onset of bipolar II disorder more strongly than other disorders, including panic disorder, alcohol dependence, and pain disorder [3].

These data converge with those of other studies in Faedda et al.'s [2] review reporting the evidence of a range of psychopathological symptoms and behavioral changes proposed as prodrome potentially leading to bipolar disorder. The association of anxiety disorders with prospectively observed bipolar disorder was confirmed by several other studies [4–8]. Such a predictive association was powerful with separation anxiety and early-onset fearful panic attacks [7], a finding also confirmed among adults with bipolar I in the NESARC study [9].

Overall, these studies indicate an association between anxiety disorders (separation anxiety, social anxiety disorder, and early-onset panic attacks) and disruptive behavior disorders (ADHD, conduct disorder) with the later development of bipolar disorder.

In other words, prodromal features extend well beyond development from affective precursors of the bipolar spectrum, with the evidence of evolution from subsyndromal and syndromal anxiety to bipolar disorder. In summary, there is evidence from the literature review of the development of bipolar disorder from a range of psychopathological loading, specifically including separation anxiety. Specifically, according to Faedda et al.'s [2] reappraisal of the evidence, there is an association between SAD and bipolar subtype: SAD predicts bipolar I and II disorder but not major depression. In addition, subsyndromal separation anxiety is predictive of bipolar II disorder but not of bipolar I or major depression. Examining prospectively observed cases reported in the literature, Faedda et al. [2] report that subthreshold or syndromal separation anxiety predicted the first onset of bipolar II disorder more strongly than other disorders, including panic attacks, alcohol dependence, and panic disorder.

Thus, bipolar disorder is often preceded by clinical risk factors such as anxiety and disruptive behavior symptoms and disorders. Further evaluation of the predictive value and contributions of such specific clinical risk factors, including separation anxiety, in the later development of bipolar disorder, can help identify populations at increased risk, guide timely and better-targeted interventions, and perhaps reduce the morbidity and mortality and improve treatment response and outcome in bipolar disorder.

1.1 Co-occurring Separation Anxiety and Bipolar Disorder in Adulthood

Data on the relationships between separation anxiety symptoms and adult bipolar disorder are scant. The most consistent hypothesis in the literature remains that early separation anxiety disorder (SAD) is specifically linked to the risk of panic disorder (PD) in adulthood [10, 11]. With few exceptions, earlier retrospective studies supported the SAD-PD hypothesis [12] and links between SAD and mood disorders [13]. However, other authors did not support an exclusive link between separation anxiety and the later development of panic disorder [13, 14]. For example, evidence concluding that there is a specific association between separation anxiety and mood dysregulation comes primarily from studies in which PD patients were compared with healthy controls, which cannot confirm specificity [15]. Other studies using controls affected by other mental disorders have argued against specificity or confirmed specificity of a SAD-later PD link only for females. Lipsitz et al. [16] suggested that SAD might be a vulnerability marker for multiple anxiety disorders rather than for PD alone. This has been corroborated by a series of other studies summarized by Wehry et al. [17]. A more recent 7.4-year follow-up of children who had received treatment for anxiety disorders reported that children with prior SAD had, compared to those with other anxiety diagnoses, more anxiety disorders in general but not specifically PD [18]. Data from the Early Developmental Stage of Psychopathology (EDSP) study provides compelling evidence on the link between SAD and bipolar disorders [19]. The study conducted in Germany on 3021 patients from adolescence to adulthood (14–24 years) reported approximately equal rates of a childhood history of SAD in patients with PD (51%) and in patients with bipolar disorders. This important prospective study provided evidence that argues against a unique relationship between SA disorder and the specificity of developing later PD. Therefore, it broadened the range of associations/risks and/or prospective overlaps between separation anxiety and different domains of psychopathology.

In a recent paper [13] almost 20% of a sample of 100 bipolar patients and 50% of the subgroup with comorbid anxiety disorders had a history of SAD. Given the high rate of PD preceding the onset of bipolar disorder, the authors assumed that SAD could also be considered a prodromal condition in the longitudinal course of BD [15]. From this perspective, consistent with the EDSP study mentioned above [20], there can be a progression from SAD to PD to bipolar disorder.

Several authors support the hypothesis that early separation anxiety is a general vulnerability factor, increasing the risk of developing anxiety and mood disorders in adulthood. Lewinsohn et al. [21], for example, in a large sample of young individuals, found that major depression (MDD) was significantly more likely to follow simple phobia and separation anxiety than PD [22, 23]. Even in a cohort of elderly medical patients 3.5% of individuals were found to have significant separation anxiety symptoms [24]. These individuals had a greater frequency of lifetime affective or anxiety disorders than those with less severe separation anxiety symptoms. Silove et al. [25, 26] demonstrated in carefully conducted epidemiological studies that a substantial proportion of individuals suffering from panic disorder have primary separation anxiety disorder followed by secondary panic attacks. Silove et al. also demonstrated that adult separation anxiety disorder and agoraphobia are distinct constructs with different clinical manifestations that are often not easily disentangled [27]. They also found that separation anxiety in adulthood has links with the bipolar spectrum [28]. Unfortunately, the nature of this link, particularly the chronological relationship between the onset of these conditions, is unclear.

Some argue that comorbid anxiety disorders may account for separation anxiety symptoms in bipolar patients. For example, Lipsitz et al. [16] compared the prevalence of childhood SA in patients with only one anxiety disorder (PD, social phobia, or OCD) and patients with the same disorder plus additional anxiety disorders. The authors reported a significant linear trend, with higher rates of childhood SA corresponding to higher numbers of comorbid disorders. Unfortunately, replication data in bipolar patients with multiple anxiety comorbidities are unavailable, a true hole in the anxious attachment/separation anxiety outcome literature. Thus far, it is not easy to find a linear association between SA, the number of comorbid anxiety disorders, and the connection with the development of bipolar spectrum. Cross-sectional multiple anxiety disorders are associated with bipolar disorder, more severe psychopathology and abuse of stimulants. Unfortunately, these studies did not evaluate separation anxiety disorder, probably because until recently, it was not acknowledged to be among the anxiety disorders that affect adults [29–31].

Notwithstanding, clinical impression, corroborated by clinical experience with adult patients with separation anxiety, suggests reciprocal influences between separation anxiety and numerous signs and symptoms of bipolarity. Most clinical reports are unclear about whether separation anxiety may reflect an underlying attachment dysregulation as aspects of the same developmental, attachment-derived relational phenomena [32]. They could also be different aspects of the same syndrome, similar to what is likely to happen, in some cases, between the reaction to abandonment in borderline personality disorder and bipolar disorder [33].

Two findings from our previous studies [34, 35] suggest a potential biological link between SA and Bipolar Disorder (BD). First, we found a stronger correlation between adult SA and a history of SA during childhood in bipolar patients than in patients with PD without comorbid bipolar disorder. Second, using regression analysis, we found that the presence of adult SA was predictive of earlier onset BD. In other words, separation anxiety is likely to contribute to characterizing BD beyond the classical differentiation into bipolar I and II subtypes [36]. Further research is needed to better characterize factors contributing to the timing of onset and/or persistence of syndromal or subthreshold SAD from childhood into adulthood and comorbidity profiles. Insights like these would inform the treatment development work needed to establish more targeted and effective preventive and clinical interventions. The paucity of clinical research in this area contrasts with the clinical impression that these two domains, namely bipolarity and sensitivity to separation, often coexist in the same individual and tend to manifest themselves in a variety of ways, depending on multiple factors (see Table 1).

One reason researchers and clinicians connect childhood separation anxiety exclusively with the development of adult anxiety disorders may be that manifestations of separation anxiety vary across the lifespan during development, complicating its presentation.

Notwithstanding, some straightforward suggestions of continuity of SA from childhood to adulthood were already advanced by Donald Klein [39], and reappraised by Ellis [27]. These authors hypothesized a biological model in which some children are genetically predisposed to react to separations with a response of overwhelming anxiety—and that this oversensitive scanning mechanism continues through adulthood. Here, data from the literature are not consistent. Klein strongly

Table 1 Distinct features of mood spectrum dysregulations in depressed patients and potential additive effects of separation anxiety symptoms or disorder on individuals' relationships (adapted from refs. [29, 30, 37])

Mood dysregulated traits	Separation anxiety symptoms or disorder[a]
Mood- rapid changes from happiness to sadness with and without knowing why	Uncertainty about the stability of the relationship
Frequent up and downs in mood with or without apparent cause	Tendency to emphasize insecurity aspects of relationships
Feelings are rather easily hurt	Minimal arguments solicit feelings of abandonment
The future looks dark sometimes	Pessimistic view of the relationship
Racing thoughts	Abnormal efforts to focus on the relationship.
Abnormal sleep pattern because of worry what happened during the day	Ruminating about relationship
Feeling disgruntled	Anger when thinking about own relationship

[a]In adults separation anxiety might be evident in the context of intimate relationship with spouse, partner, and significant relative(s) or close friend(s) or pets (see [38])

supported the idea of a direct link between SA and panic disorder/agoraphobia. Other authors suggested that childhood separation anxiety may not be related to panic disorder per se but may be a risk factor that predisposes patients to develop an agoraphobic avoidance pattern once panic disorder has begun [40].

The question remains controversial. In this regard, it is noteworthy that the DSM-5 has included adult separation anxiety disorder in Section 2 of the book within anxiety disorders, thereby acknowledging that adulthood can be a period in which separation anxiety may appear. Thus, it may play a role across the lifespan. What is unclear is whether childhood separation anxiety disorder usually persists into adulthood, suggesting continuities between CSAD and ASAD or whether it is more common that ASAD occurs as an onset of separation anxiety symptoms in adulthood [41]. In either case, the "continuity hypothesis" and "adult-onset hypothesis" cannot explain what determines separation anxiety becomes clinically relevant or, in some cases, debilitating for the individuals. From this perspective, the clinical nature of separation anxiety can shed light on its potential role as a prodrome or risk factor for bipolar disorders and vice versa. The onset of a bipolar syndrome may amplify the impact of separation anxiety on an individual's functioning [42]. In other cases, it is separation anxiety disorder that makes a bipolar diathesis more clinically meaningful, especially in the relational area than it would have been without the separation anxiety component.

Separation anxiety has been variously described in developmental research and attachment theory [43]. Distress upon separation from one's close attachment figure(s) is the developmental norm during early childhood. It is an evolutionarily adaptive mechanism designed to keep the defenseless child close to his adult caregiver(s). Only when separation distress becomes prolonged, excessive, and developmentally inappropriate or impairing is a psychiatric diagnosis typically made. The estimated prevalence of childhood separation anxiety disorder in the general population is 4%. An adult form of this syndrome is now listed in DSM-5. However, some researchers in the field note that even when a distinct constellation of SA symptoms is present, clinicians do not usually make a diagnosis [44]. Silove et al. [44] note that, from a clinical perspective, Bowlby's developmental model of agoraphobia provided a clinical elaboration of this common clinical phenomenon. He proposed that if high levels of SA persisted into later years, it manifests as typical symptoms of agoraphobia [45]. According to this model, symptoms such as carrying transitional objects, reliance on phobic companions, and the preference for staying at home (as a symbol of a secure base or a substitution for a stabilizing attachment relationship) reveal the underlying separation anxiety roots of adult agoraphobia.

The importance of adult-onset separation anxiety disorder is indicated in that 20–40% of adult patients with mood and anxiety disorders have been found to have symptoms of the disorder, and between one-third and one-half of these patients reported onset after 18 years of age [34, 46]. Patients with adult separation anxiety disorder experience high levels of functional impairment and show a poor response to conventional treatments used for other anxiety subtypes [47, 48].

Despite the importance of the Silove et al. [28] study, there are still inadequate epidemiologic data focusing on separation anxiety disorder across the lifespan. A longitudinal study commencing in childhood recorded a 5% lifetime prevalence of separation anxiety disorder by the time the cohort reached early adulthood [28]. The National Comorbidity Survey Replication in the USA found a lifetime separation anxiety disorder prevalence of 6.6% after the pediatric age-at-onset requirement was removed, with two-thirds of case subjects having onset after 17 years of age. Still, comparable data in other samples or populations have yet to be reported.

Manicavasagar et al. [49] proposed that the core symptoms of separation anxiety—that is excessive and often disabling distress in the face of actual or perceived separation from major attachment figures—might indeed persist or arise throughout adulthood. Clinical case studies indicate that adult separation anxiety represents a discrete diagnostic entity worthy of clinical attention. By its very nature, all separation anxiety, including that which presents during adulthood, occurs within an interpersonal field involving the family and close attachments, which may include pets. A pattern of collusion, in willing, or similarly burdened close attachment figures, may arise in which the person with SAD, the family, and therefore the clinician all underestimate the role of SAD symptoms as a source of dysfunction in the patient. This is the so-called ego-syntonicity of SAD [44, 50]. Definitional symptom overlap, particularly between agoraphobia and SAD, may further confound the picture. Moreover, SAD may also occur in relation to the disruptions and losses associated with other severe mental disorders, such as bipolar disorder. In these contexts, the mood-related symptoms will often overshadow those of separation anxiety, which, as a consequence, will go undetected, even though they add to the person's overall disability.

1.2 The Mixture of the Bipolar Spectrum with Separation Anxiety Disorder: The Case of Cyclothymia

Severe adult forms of separation anxiety may present in various ways—including suicidal behaviors [51] in response to actual or threatened separations. This is not noted in the DSM-5 criteria.

Monica, a 24-year old, unmarried woman presented with a history of "moodiness" since she was 14. The patient said one day she would be "high like a kite" and the next day she would stay in bed. Her moods changed every few days, sometimes daily, but she was able to finish high school and worked as a shop assistant for high-end fashion brands; she was known for her traits of dependability and independence. Since childhood, she remembers she got anxious when her parents left her alone even for a short time, and often had scary fantasies of abandonment and worried that harm would befall them. She had nightmares about this persisting to adulthood. At age 18 she started having more protracted depressive episodes twice yearly, in the autumn and in the spring, lasting for 3–4 weeks. She described that the one in the autumn was characterized by sleeping too much and overeating, and the one in the spring by "a peculiar mixture of physical slowing, irritability, mental restlessness, and hypersexuality". She had received numerous antidepressants for "depression", to no avail. Her response to these was generally disappointing, indeed she insisted that her "PMS" got worse from medication. She was prescribed an SSRI, and after 3 weeks she felt suddenly energized—her mind "running 200 miles a minute"—she could literally "climb the mountain" where she lived, was overconfident, and slept with several men daily, the entire episode lasting 2 weeks. The patient had lived in different places since she was 18; she would simply take off, unsatisfied with the place or the people. Over the past year she was hospitalized once because, after a minimal argument, she was "terrified by the possibility of being dumped by my fiancé" and hurt herself with cigarette butts and hair curlers. Family history was significant for bipolar disorder in that the mother, described by the patient as "a flamboyant bitch", had been divorced four times, and had many lovers well into her 70 s; a maternal aunt, diagnosed manic-depressive, died in a mental institution. Her biological father drank alcohol excessively. Mental status examination revealed a young woman who complained that she was plump, with a distinctive flair in her attire. She used rich and dramatic expressions in describing her life and moods. Although her facial expression displayed bright affect, she said if lightning struck her dead, she would thank God. She spoke about her "utter failure with romantic relationships, despite initiating each of them with enthusiasm and excitement." "I always get clingy with my partner and finally it turns against me". She described episodes of extreme anxiety and discomfort when confronted by thoughts related to separation from a significant person, for instance, her grandmother or her sister or mother.

She said her sister was like her, "only worse because she uses all kinds of substances, especially uppers". The patient concluded the interview by saying that she was a "borderline person". It is noteworthy that this patient at the trait level (looking only at SCID II for example) would meet the criteria for "borderline personality"—which was indeed the diagnosis she carried in her past medical records—yet she suffers discrete mood episodes with a specific seasonal pattern; spontaneous hypomanic episodes were of short duration, never meeting the DSM-5 threshold of 4 days, she had a hypomanic response to SSRIs, placing her in the so-called "Bipolar III" category (F31.89/cyclothymia). However, Monica always suffered from waxing-and-waning separation anxiety that carried with it dramatic consequences in intimate relationships. Her spring "depressions" would be better described as depressive mixed states, although again they fall below the DSM-5 threshold. The family history points to a strong bipolar diathesis, indicating that her primary mood disorder is likely Bipolar II or III. Clinically, therefore, it would make sense to consider this patient as continuously shifting between cyclothymia and major depression with co-occurrence of separation anxiety disorder.

The clinical case described above highlights the impact of separation anxiety across the bipolar spectrum. Such an interaction, for instance, is quite evident in patients described with cyclothymic depression (see case vignette). Akiskal and Pinto [52] report that these patients have moderately to severely impairing recurrent major depression, interspersed with hypomanic periods of a few days duration without marked impairment: although the elated mood colors the behavior, confidence, and optimism, and judgment is relatively preserved compared to full-blown mania. Cassano et al. [29, 30] adopted a more unitary approach to bipolarity and proposed the inclusion of different subtypes of bipolar disorder into the same mood disorder spectrum. Within this framework, the cyclic course of the disease may involve periods of significant dysfunction and serious suicide attempts. Mood lability may be a trait characteristic in such patients and need not manifest in DSM-5 hypomanic periods (see Table 1).

It is noteworthy that, except for the first two traits, mood lability is in a depressive direction. The underlying cyclic mood changes permit normal to supra-normal periods of functioning. A not-inconsiderable number of these patients can rebound from their difficult periods to attain new romantic or occupational status. Thus, if chronic separation anxiety is present as a backdrop, it may become prominent as a preoccupying syndrome that contributes to current dysfunction depending on the person's mood state and fluctuations, typically disappearing during hyperthymic periods and exacerbating during depressive phases. The fact that SAD symptoms can come and go during adulthood and that broad mood states can for periods overshadow them may, in part, contribute to why SAD has gone relatively unnoticed in adults for so long. As described in Clinical Case 2, in some cases, mood stabilization commonly reveals that SAD is a major factor affecting an individual's difficulties with psychosocial functioning.

According to the DSM-5 schema, many bipolar patients do not meet the strict DSM-5 criteria for bipolar II or I. For example, patients with short duration of hypomania often have a recurrent pattern of periods of excitement, followed by mini depressions, thereby fulfilling the criteria for cyclothymic disorder. Other individuals have hypomanic episodes of short duration (2–3 days) and major depressive episodes. From a longitudinal perspective, these individuals have a lifetime history of one or more major depressive episodes and never met the full criteria for a manic or hypomanic episode but have experienced two or more episodes of short duration hypomania that meet the full symptomatic criteria for a hypomanic episode but that only last for 2–3 days. The episodes of hypomanic symptoms do not overlap in time with the major depressive episodes, so the disturbance does not meet the criteria for a major depressive episode with mixed features. When a major depressive episode is superimposed on this baseline, the diagnosis of bipolar disorder may be entirely missed because the instability in the life of a cyclothymic may be such that they appear to meet criteria for Axis II cluster B personality disorders at the trait level and wind up carrying this diagnosis [53].

In brief, these patients are likely to be labeled as "borderline" rather than as affectively ill [54]. Within this framework, the role of separation anxiety disorder may be crucial in shaping the clinical picture (see Table 1). Looking at these patients through the lens of separation anxiety, adults with a diagnosis of separation anxiety disorder report extreme anxiety about separations from major attachment figures (partner, children, or parents), fear that harm would befall those close to them, and the perceived need to maintain proximity to them. These symptoms may affect the individual's behavior and lead to severe impairment in social relationships and distortions in life choices from this degree of attachment insecurity.

It is important to distinguish between symptoms of separation anxiety and dependent personality traits, which may also occur in patients with bipolar disorders [55]. Dependency is a pervasive and indiscriminate tendency to rely excessively on others. In contrast, separation anxiety refers to a limited array of concerns about the proximity and safety of key attachment figures [56]. Furthermore, there is clinical evidence that feelings of abandonment and severe SA symptoms are not rare in patients with bipolar disorder (BD), especially in connection with situations, either objective or perceived, that threaten their bond and proximity to significant others. The Pisa group conducted research in this framework [56] in a sample of about 500 adult outpatients. Pini and colleagues aimed to evaluate the severity and frequency of SA symptoms, as well as the frequency of childhood and adult separation anxiety disorders separately, among patients with bipolar disorder as compared to patients with panic disorder (PD) (without comorbid MDD), major depression (MDD) (without comorbid PD), and a group of healthy individuals (HC) with no psychiatric disorders. The relationship between age at the onset of bipolar disorder and of separation anxiety was also explored with the Structured Clinical Interview assessed separation anxiety for Separation Anxiety—Childhood section (SCI-SAS-C) and the Structured Clinical Interview for Separation Anxiety—Adult section (SCI-SAS-A) [57]. Results showed a linear correlation between both the SCI-SAS-C total score and the SCI-SAS-A total score and the age of onset of bipolar disorder. A linear regression was performed to predict age at onset of BD as a dependent variable, using SCI-SAS-C and SCI-SAS-A total scores as dependent variables and controlling for age, sex, and panic disorder comorbidity. These analyses showed that both SCI-SAS-C ($p < 0.02$) and SCI-SAS-A ($p < 0.0001$) total scores were significantly predictive of age at the onset of bipolar disorder. In particular, the presence of SA during adulthood was associated with an earlier onset of bipolar disorder.

Further investigation into the presence and effects of separation anxiety in adults with bipolar disorder is warranted by these solid data. Our research group conducted several studies exploring separation anxiety symptoms in adult bipolar disorder patients. Our research group, about 10 years after the first report on separation anxiety and bipolar disorder, returned to this exploration [58]. This study aimed to investigate the prevalence and correlates of separation anxiety disorder among patients with PD and whether the presence of separation anxiety disorder was associated with frank diagnoses of mood disorders or symptoms, in particular, bipolar spectrum symptoms (not necessarily reaching the threshold for bipolar I or II). Mood spectrum symptoms were assessed with the Mood Spectrum Self-Report Instrument (MOODS-SR), which was developed and validated by an international collaborative group of researchers (Spectrum Project) [29, 30]. Here, we shall briefly describe the MOODS-SR. The MOODS-SR assesses lifetime mood spectrum symptoms, including prodromal, residual, atypical, and subclinical characteristics. MOODS-SR provides a rating for significant affective symptoms but also identifies and rates atypical and mild symptomatic manifestations as expressions of subclinical conditions. The sum of the scores on the three manic domains (mood, energy, cognition) constitutes the "manic component" (62 items), and that of the three depressive domains includes the "depressive component" (63 items).

In Gesi et al.'s [58] study, of the 235 adult outpatients with panic disorder, 125 (53.2%) were categorized as having adult separation anxiety disorder and 110 (46.8%) as not. Groups did not differ regarding the onset of panic disorder, the lifetime prevalence of obsessive-compulsive disorder, social phobia, simple phobia, BD I and II, or major depressive disorder (MDD). Patients with both PD and SAD showed higher levels of lifetime mood spectrum symptoms compared to PD patients without SAD. Specifically, SAD subjects showed higher total and manic/hypomanic component scores on the MOODS-SR than patients without SAD, even accounting for the effects of age, gender, the presence of lifetime comorbidity with frank bipolar disorder and major depression, and severity of PD symptoms. These findings are potentially like previous data showing a strong correlation between SAD symptoms and lifetime mood symptoms of both polarities in a sample of patients with anxiety or mood disorders, and 23% had complicated grief as an adjunctive condition [59].

In Gesi et al.'s study [58], it is possible that PD patients who also show features of adult SAD are more vulnerable to experiencing mood symptoms. The important distinction may be that, despite not reporting a higher rate of lifetime frank mood diagnoses, adult separation anxiety is correlated with greater lifetime mood spectrum symptoms, particularly in the manic/hypomanic domain. These data might be consistent with previous postulates that constellations of early phobic anxiety, including adult SAD, could be linked to subthreshold bipolar spectrum features such as mood lability or cyclothymia.

A further possibility is that adult SAD is a marker for PD severity. This hypothesis is consistent with the greater severity of PD that we found in the adult SAD group. That finding, together with the higher scores reported by adult SAD subjects on the MOODS-SR, might be interpreted as indicating that these patients experience a greater level of emotional lability of a generic type as a lifelong tendency, including a tendency to more severe panic and mood symptoms, potentially stemming from early separation anxiety or attachment difficulties. However, our results also show that adult SAD subjects score higher on the MOODS-SR, even controlling for PD symptom severity (evaluated with the PDSS), suggesting a specific vulnerability to affective spectrum symptoms. Further studies that consider other possible confounding factors (including, for example, the presence of agoraphobia) will help disentangle the pattern of vulnerability to panic and anxiety as opposed to mood spectrum symptoms among patients with comorbid PD and adult SAD.

Interestingly, in Gesi et al.'s study [58], separation anxiety was shown to predict poorer responses to psychological and psychopharmacological PD treatments. We hypothesize that this differential treatment response could be partly due to greater mood spectrum bipolar symptoms in persons with separation anxiety disorder.

The lack of robust measures of temperamental characteristics and Axis II disorders did not allow us to investigate whether associations between adult SAD and mood spectrum symptoms might be mediated by underlying characterological disturbances. In addition, although we found some critical associations between adult SAD and mood symptoms, we could not determine the direction of causality. Further longitudinal studies are necessary to elucidate this relationship. Despite these limitations, our results suggested that, in a clinic sample in which those with current comorbidity with frank mood disorders are removed, subjects with both PD and adult SAD had a distinct profile characterized by greater lifetime bipolar spectrum symptoms, greater severity of panic symptoms, and history of early adult SAD compared with subjects with PD alone or PD with other comorbidities. This profile of comorbid SAD and PD may explain the high levels of functional impairment and resistance to conventional treatments found among these patients. SAD's inherent dysregulation of attachment relationships, with profound implications for SAD patients' common difficulty establishing adequate social support [60], establishing a trusting relationship with a psychiatrist may be fractured for these people, further straining care. Further studies are warranted to investigate the possible mediating factors in these relationships.

In summary, the data discussed in this chapter appear to be preliminary grounds for investigating further the possibility that separation anxiety may deserve greater recognition in adults with bipolar disorder. It would be interesting in future studies to investigate to what extent SA may also be specifically associated with different forms or subtypes of bipolar disorder. Furthermore, such research might also help elucidate factors that contribute to adult-onset and/or persistence of syndromal or subthreshold SAD from childhood into adulthood, either occurring singly or comorbid with other psychiatric disorders. Insights like these would inform treatment development work needed to establish effective preventive and clinical interventions for this disorder.

References

1. Faedda GL, Marangoni C, Serra G, Salvatore P, Sani G, Vázquez GH, Tondo L, Girardi P, Baldessarini RJ, Koukopoulos A. Precursors of bipolar disorders: a systematic literature review of prospective studies. J Clin Psychiatry. 2015;76(5):614–24. https://doi.org/10.4088/JCP.13r08900.
2. Faedda GL, Serra G, Marangoni C, Salvatore P, Sani G, Vázquez GH, Tondo L, Girardi P, Baldessarini RJ, Koukopoulos A. Clinical risk factors for bipolar disorders: a systematic

review of prospective studies. J Affect Disord. 2014;168:314–21. https://doi.org/10.1016/j.jad.2014.07.013. Epub 2014 Jul 18
3. Brückl TM, Wittchen HU, Höfler M, Pfister H, Schneider S, Lieb R. Childhood separation anxiety and the risk of subsequent psychopathology: results from a community study. Psychother Psychosom. 2007;76:47–56.
4. Homish GG, Marshall D, Dubovsky SL, Leonard K. Predictors of later bipolar disorder in patients with subthreshold symptoms. J Affect Disord. 2013;144:129–33.
5. Johnson JG, Cohen P, Brook JS. Associations between bipolar disorder and other psychiatric disorders during adolescence and early adulthood: a community-based longitudinal investigation. Am J Psychiatry. 2000;157(10):1679–81. https://doi.org/10.1176/appi.ajp.157.10.1679.
6. Grant BF, Goldstein RB, Chou SP, Huang B, Stinson FS, Dawson DA, Saha TD, Smith SM, Pulay AJ, Pickering RP, Ruan WJ, Compton WM. Sociodemographic and psychopathologic predictors of first incidence of DSM-IV substance use, mood and anxiety disorders: results from the Wave2 National Epidemiologic Survey on Alcohol and Related Conditions. Mol Psychiatry. 2009;14:1051–66.
7. Kinley DJ, Walker JR, Enns MW, Sareen J. Panic attacks as a risk for later psychopathology: results from a nationally representative survey. Depress Anxiety. 2011;28(5):412–9. https://doi.org/10.1002/da.20809.
8. Chou KL, Mackenzie CS, Liang K, Sareen J. Three-year incidence and predictors of first-onset of DSM-IV mood, anxiety, and substance use disorders in older adults: results from wave 2 of the National Epidemiologic Survey on alcohol and related conditions. J Clin Psychiatry. 2011;72(2):144–55. https://doi.org/10.4088/JCP.09m05618gry.
9. Goldstein BI, Levitt AJ. Prevalence and correlates of bipolar I disorder among adults with primary youth-onset anxiety disorders. J Affect Disord. 2007;103:187–95.
10. Gittelman-Klein R. Is panic disorder associated with childhood separation anxiety disorder? Clin Neuropharmacol. 1995;18(7–14):4.
11. Kossowsky J, Pfaltz MC, Schneider S, Taeymans J, Locher C, Gaab J. The separation anxiety hypothesis of panic disorder revisited: a meta-analysis. Am J Psychiatry. 2013;170(7):768–81. https://doi.org/10.1176/appi.ajp.2012.12070893.
12. Battaglia M, Bertella S, Politi E, Bernardeschi L, Perna G, Gabriele A, Bellodi L. Age of onset of panic disorder: influence of familial liability to the disease and of childhood separation anxiety disorder. Am J Psychiatry. 1995;152:1362–4.
13. Caricasole V, Di Bernardo I, Varinelli A, Galimberti C, Zanello R, Bosi M, Ketter TA, Viganò CA, Dell'Osso B. Anxiety disorders anticipate the diagnosis of bipolar disorder in comorbid patients: findings from an Italian tertiary clinic. J Affect Disord. 2019;257:376–81. https://doi.org/10.1016/j.jad.2019.07.033. Epub 2019 Jul 5
14. Silove D, He Y, Ferrand M, Scott K. Separation anxiety disorder. In: Scott K, De Jonge P, Stein D, Kessler R, editors. Mental disorders around the world: facts and figures from the WHO world mental health surveys. Cambridge: Cambridge University Press; 2018. p. 167–81. https://doi.org/10.1017/9781316336168.012.
15. Tasdemir A, Tamam L, Keskin N, Evlice YE. Assessment of co-morbidity of adult separation anxiety in patients with bipolar disorder. Nord J Psychiatry. 2016;70(2):93–102. https://doi.org/10.3109/08039488.2015.1053098.
16. Lipsitz JD, Martin LY, Mannuzza S, Chapman TF, Liebowitz MR, Klein DF, Fyer AJ. Childhood separation anxiety disorder in patients with adult anxiety disorders. Am J Psychiatry. 1994;151:927–9.
17. Wehry AM, Beesdo-Baum K, Hennelly MM, Connolly SD, Strawn JR. Assessment and treatment of anxiety disorders in children and adolescents. Curr Psychiatry Rep. 2015;17(7):52. https://doi.org/10.1007/s11920-015-0591-z.
18. Kossowsky J, Wilhelm FH, Roth WT, Schneider S. Separation anxiety disorder in children: disorder-specific responses to experimental separation from the mother. J Child Psychol Psychiatry. 2012;53(2):178–87. https://doi.org/10.1111/j.1469-7610.2011.02465.x. Epub 2011 Sep 16

19. Wittchen H-U, Perkonigg A, Lachner G, Nelson CB. Early developmental stages of psychopathology study (EDSP): objectives and design. Eur Addict Res. 1998;4:18–27.
20. Beesdo-Baum K, Knappe S, Asselmann E, et al. The 'Early developmental stages of psychopathology (EDSP) study': a 20-year review of methods and findings. Soc Psychiatry Psychiatr Epidemiol. 2015;50(6):851–66. https://doi.org/10.1007/s00127-015-1062-x.
21. Lewinsohn PM, Holm-Denoma JM, Small JW, Seeley JR, Joiner TE Jr. Separation anxiety disorder in childhood as a risk factor for future mental illness. J Am Acad Child Adolesc Psychiatry. 2008;47(5):548–55. https://doi.org/10.1097/CHI.0b013e31816765e7.
22. Lewinsohn PM, Rohde P, Seeley JR. Major depressive disorder in older adolescents: prevalence, risk factors, and clinical implications. Clin Psychol Rev. 1998;18(7):765–94. https://doi.org/10.1016/s0272-7358(98)00010-5.
23. Elbay RY, Görmez A, Kılıç A, Avcı SH. Separation anxiety disorder among outpatients with major depressive disorder: prevalence and clinical correlates. Compr Psychiatry. 2021;105:152219. https://doi.org/10.1016/j.comppsych.2020.152219.
24. Wijeratne C, Manicavasagar V. Separation anxiety in the elderly. J Anxiety Disord. 2003;17(6):695–702. https://doi.org/10.1016/s0887-6185(02)00239-6.
25. Silove D, Liddell B, Rees S, et al. Effects of recurrent violence on post-traumatic stress disorder and severe distress in conflict-affected Timor-Leste: a 6-year longitudinal study. Lancet Glob Health. 2014;2(5):e293–300. https://doi.org/10.1016/S2214-109X(14)70196-2.
26. Silove D, Ivancic L, Rees S, Bateman-Steel C, Steel Z. Clustering of symptoms of mental disorder in the mediumterm following conflict: an epidemiological study in Timor-Leste. Psychiatry Res. 2014;219(2):341–6. https://doi.org/10.1016/j.psychres.2014.05.043.
27. Ellis EM. Adult agoraphobia and childhood separation anxiety: using children's literature to understand the link. Am J Psychother. 1990;44(3):433–44. https://doi.org/10.1176/appi.psychotherapy.1990.44.3.433.
28. Silove D, Alonso J, Bromet E, Gruber M, Sampson N, Scott K, Andrade L, Benjet C, Caldas de Almeida JM, De Girolamo G, de Jonge P, Demyttenaere K, Fiestas F, Florescu S, Gureje O, He Y, Karam E, Lepine JP, Murphy S, Villa-Posada J, Zarkov Z, Kessler RC. Pediatric-onset and adult-onset separation anxiety disorder across countries in the World Mental Health Survey. Am J Psychiatry. 2015;172(7):647–56. https://doi.org/10.1176/appi.ajp.2015.14091185. Epub 2015 Jun 5
29. Cassano GB, Pini S, Saettoni M, Dell'Osso L. Multiple anxiety disorder comorbidity in patients with mood spectrum disorders with psychotic features. Am J Psychiatry. 1999;156(3):474–6. https://doi.org/10.1176/ajp.156.3.474.
30. Cassano GB, Dell'Osso L, Frank E, Miniati M, Fagiolini A, Shear K, Pini S, Maser J. The bipolar spectrum: a clinical reality in search of diagnostic criteria and an assessment methodology. J Affect Disord. 1999;54(3):319–28. https://doi.org/10.1016/s0165-0327(98)00158-x.
31. Pini S, Cassano GB, Simonini E, Savino M, Russo A, Montgomery SA. Prevalence of anxiety disorders comorbidity in bipolar depression, unipolar depression and dysthymia. J Affect Disord. 1997;42(2–3):145–53.
32. Milrod B, Keefe JR, Choo TH, Arnon S, Such S, Lowell A, Neria Y, Markowitz JC. Separation anxiety in PTSD: a pilot study of mechanisms in patients undergoing IPT. Depress Anxiety. 2020;37(4):386–95. https://doi.org/10.1002/da.23003. Epub 2020 Feb 25
33. Paris J. Differential diagnosis of borderline personality disorder. Psychiatr Clin North Am. 2018;41(4):575–82. https://doi.org/10.1016/j.psc.2018.07.001.
34. Pini S, Abelli M, Shear KM, et al. Frequency and clinical correlates of adult separation anxiety in a sample of 508 outpatients with mood and anxiety disorders. Acta Psychiatr Scand. 2010;122:40–6.
35. Costa B, Pini S, Baldwin DS, et al. Oxytocin receptor and G-protein polymorphisms in patients with depression and separation anxiety. J Affect Disord. 2017;218:365–73.
36. Fagiolini A, Frank E, Rucci P, Cassano GB, Turkin S, Kupfer DJ. Mood and anxiety spectrum as a means to identify clinically relevant subtypes of bipolar I disorder. Bipolar Disord. 2007;9(5):462–7. https://doi.org/10.1111/j.1399-5618.2007.00443.x.

37. Cassano GB, Rucci P, Benvenuti A, Miniati M, Calugi S, Maggi L, et al. The role of psychomotor activation in discriminating unipolar from bipolar disorders: a classification-tree analysis. J Clin Psychiatry. 2012;73:22–8.
38. Shear MK, Cassano GB, Frank E, Rucci P, Rotondo A, Fagiolini A. The panic-agoraphobic spectrum: development, description, and clinical significance. Psychiatr Clin North Am. 2002;25(4):739–56.
39. Klein DF. Anxiety reconceptualized. Compr Psychiatry. 1980;21:411–27.
40. Zitrin CM, Ross DC. Early separation anxiety and adult agoraphobia. J Nerv Ment Dis. 1988;176(10):621–5. https://doi.org/10.1097/00005053-198810000-00007.
41. Manicavasagar V, Marnane C, Pini S, et al. Adult separation anxiety disorder: a disorder comes of age. Curr Psychiatry Rep. 2010;12(4):290–7.
42. Pini S, Abelli M, Mauri M, Muti M, Iazzetta P, Banti S, Cassano GB. Clinical correlates and significance of separation anxiety in patients with bipolar disorder. Bipolar Disord. 2005;7(4):370–6. https://doi.org/10.1111/j.1399-5618.2005.00216.x.
43. Main M. Revisiting the founder of attachment theory: memories and informal reflections. Attach Hum Dev. 2021;23(4):468–80. https://doi.org/10.1080/14616734.2021.1918447. Epub 2021 May 10
44. Silove D, Manicavasagar V, Pini S. Can separation anxiety disorder escape its attachment to childhood? World Psychiatry. 2016;15(2):113–5. https://doi.org/10.1002/wps.20336.
45. Bowlby J. Attachment and loss, vol. 2. New York: Basic Books; 1999/1973.
46. Silove DM, Marnane CL, Wagner R, et al. The prevalence and correlates of adult separation anxiety disorder in an anxiety clinic. BMC Psychiatry. 2010;10:21.
47. Bögels SM, Knappe S, Clark LA. Adult separation anxiety disorder in DSM-5. Clin Psychol Rev. 2013;33(5):663–74. https://doi.org/10.1016/j.cpr.2013.03.006.
48. Milrod B, Markowitz JC, Gerber AJ, et al. Childhood separation anxiety and the pathogenesis and treatment of adult anxiety. Am J Psychiatry. 2014;171(1):34–43. https://doi.org/10.1176/appi.ajp.2013.13060781.
49. Manicavasagar V, Silove D, Curtis J, Wagner R. Continuities of separation anxiety from early life into adulthood. J Anxiety Disord. 2000;14(1):1–18. https://doi.org/10.1016/s0887-6185(99)00029-8.
50. Milrod B. An epidemiological contribution to clinical understanding of anxiety. Am J Psychiatr. 2015;172:601–2.
51. Pini S, Abelli M, Costa B, et al. Separation anxiety and measures of suicide risk among patients with mood and anxiety disorders. J Clin Psychiatry. 2021;82(2):20m13299. Published 2021 Mar 16. https://doi.org/10.4088/JCP.20m13299.
52. Akiskal HS, Pinto O. The evolving bipolar spectrum. Prototypes I, II, III, and IV. Psychiatr Clin North Am. 1999;22(3):517–vii. https://doi.org/10.1016/s0193-953x(05)70093-9.
53. Brieger P, Marneros A. Dysthymia and cyclothymia: historical origins and contemporary development. J Affect Disord. 1997;45(3):117–26. https://doi.org/10.1016/s0165-0327(97)00053-0.
54. Mc Elroy S, Freeman M, Akiskal HS. The mixed bipolar disorders. In: Marneros A, Angst J, editors. Bipolar disorders. Amsterdam: Kluwer Academic Publishers; 2000. p. 63–88.
55. Yao J, Xu Y, Qin Y, Liu J, Shen Y, Wang W, Chen W. Relationship between personality disorder functioning styles and the emotional states in bipolar I and II disorders. PLoS One. 2015;10(1):e0117353. https://doi.org/10.1371/journal.pone.0117353.
56. Pini S, Abelli M, Shear KM, Cardini A, Lari L, Gesi C, Muti M, Calugi S, Galderisi S, Troisi A, Bertolino A, Cassano GB. Frequency and clinical correlates of adult separation anxiety in a sample of 508 outpatients with mood and anxiety disorders. Acta Psychiatr Scand 2010 Jul;122(1):40–46. https://doi.org/10.1111/j.1600-0447.2009.01480.x. Epub 2009 Oct 13. PMID: 19824987.
57. Cyranowski JM, Shear MK, Rucci P, et al. Adult separation anxiety: psychometric properties of a new structured clinical interview. J Psychiatr Res. 2002;36(2):77–86.

58. Gesi C, Abelli M, Cardini A, Lari L, Di Paolo L, Silove D, Pini S. Separation anxiety disorder from the perspective of DSM-5: clinical investigation among subjects with panic disorder and associations with mood disorders spectrum. CNS Spectr. 2016;21(1):70–5. https://doi.org/10.1017/S1092852914000807. Epub 2015 Feb 23.
59. Pini S, Gesi C, Abelli M, Muti M, Lari L, Cardini A, Manicavasagar V, Mauri M, Cassano GB, Shear KM. The relationship between adult separation anxiety disorder and complicated grief in a cohort of 454 outpatients with mood and anxiety disorders. J Affect Disord. 2012;143(1–3):64–8. https://doi.org/10.1016/j.jad.2012.05.026. Epub 2012 Jul 23.
60. Markowitz JC, Lipsitz J, Milrod BL. A critical review of outcome research on interpersonal psychotherapy for anxiety disorders. Depress Anxiety. 2014;31(4):316–25.

The Distinction of Adult Separation Anxiety Disorder: Evidence and Uncertainty

David S. Baldwin, Laura Molteni, and Vasilios G. Masdrakis

The DSM-5 classification of mental disorders locates separation anxiety disorder within a broad group of anxiety disorders and acknowledges that its diagnosis no longer requires establishing an onset of symptoms during childhood or adolescence. In previous DSM editions, separation anxiety disorder had been included within the conditions typically first diagnosed in early life (infancy, childhood or adolescence) with the stipulation for the onset of symptoms before the age of 18 years – adults with separation anxiety symptoms could only receive a retrospective diagnosis, based on establishing an onset earlier in life. The ICD-11 takes a broadly similar approach to DSM-5, with the possibility of diagnosing an adult-onset condition and

D. S. Baldwin (✉)
Clinical and Experimental Sciences (Clinical Neuroscience), Faculty of Medicine, University of Southampton, Southampton, UK

University Department of Psychiatry and Mental Health, University of Cape Town, Cape Town, South Africa

Mood and Anxiety Disorders Service, Southern Health NHS Foundation Trust, Southampton, UK
e-mail: D.S.Baldwin@soton.ac.uk

L. Molteni
Clinical and Experimental Sciences (Clinical Neuroscience), Faculty of Medicine, University of Southampton, Southampton, UK

Luigi Sacco University Hospital, Psychiatry 2 Unit, University of Milan, Milan, Italy
e-mail: L.Molteni@soton.ac.uk

V. G. Masdrakis
Clinical and Experimental Sciences (Clinical Neuroscience), Faculty of Medicine, University of Southampton, Southampton, UK

First Department of Psychiatry, Eginition Hospital, National and Kapodistrian University of Athens Medical School, Athens, Greece
e-mail: vmasdrakis@med.uoa.gr

S. Pini, B. Milrod (eds.), *Separation Anxiety in Adulthood*,
https://doi.org/10.1007/978-3-031-37446-3_8

recognizing that the disorder can occur with or without coexisting panic attacks. The new position of separation anxiety disorder within the DSM-5 and ICD-11 derive from the unanticipated findings of multiple epidemiological studies that indicated a high prevalence of the condition in adults, often in people with an onset of characteristic symptoms after the teenage years. Increased awareness of the condition encourages further research into its psychopathology, aetiology, and treatment. This chapter reviews the clinical features and sometimes blurred boundaries of the disorder and suggests how it may be distinguished from other mental disorders in which 'separation anxiety' is also a feature.

1 Diagnosis of Separation Anxiety Disorder in Adults in DSM-5 and ICD-11

A diagnosis of 'adult-onset adult separation anxiety disorder' allows for the inclusion of individuals whose separation anxiety symptoms first appeared in adulthood, without a documented history of related symptoms during childhood. By contrast, the designation of 'childhood-onset adult separation anxiety disorder' encompasses those individuals whose symptoms had a childhood-onset and persistence into adult life [1]. Many adults with anxiety disorders have difficulties related to adverse childhood experiences and unsupportive environments, which only manifest subsequently through symptoms in adulthood. Separation anxiety disorder is considered in a similar way as these other conditions: by removing the age of onset stipulation and the need for separate juvenile and adult groups in both the DSM-5 and ICD-11, it aligns with the approach to diagnosis in other anxiety disorders [2].

In DSM-5 [3], separation anxiety disorder is characterized by developmentally inappropriate and excessive fear or anxiety concerning separation from attachment figures. Fear, anxiety, or avoidance of separation must have been present for at least 4 weeks in a child or adolescent, and 'typically' for at least 6 months in an adult. Diagnosis also requires the presence of at least three of eight features, including recurrent excessive distress when anticipating or experiencing separation and persistent and excessive worry about losing major attachment figures. This is potentially problematic, as it may be hard to distinguish fear and anxiety concerning separation from attachment figures (the characteristic feature) from excessive distress when anticipating or experiencing separation or from excessive worry about losing attachment figures (two of the supporting features). Furthermore, another two supporting features include a persistent reluctance or refusal to go out, away from home, or to school or work because of fear of separation; and persistent fear or reluctance about being alone or without major attachment figures at home or in other settings: which seems a rather tricky distinction, as the features can blur into those of agoraphobia.

The criterion of 'persistent and excessive worry about experiencing an untoward event' that causes separation from an attachment figure to be difficult can be hard to distinguish from the persistent and excessive worrying about family members that is troublesome in many patients with generalized anxiety disorder (GAD), although in GAD worries about others tend not to focus solely on separation concerns.

Moreover, the features of troubled sleep whilst being away from attachment figures, and repeated nightmares about separation seem hard to delineate from sleep disturbances in those patients with post-traumatic stress disorder (PTSD) whose trauma involved witnessing significant threats to family members.

Potential difficulties in formulating a diagnosis are not restricted to DSM-5 criteria. Similar problems were inherent in the diagnostic criteria for separation anxiety disorder in childhood, included within ICD-10 [4]. In this, at least three of eight features had to be present, including persistent and excessive worry about possible harm befalling major attachment figures and persistent and excessive worry that some untoward event will separate the child from an attachment figure (which posed something of a conundrum if the worrisome and anticipated untoward event involved harm). It can be hard to distinguish anxiety and worry about harm potentially befalling an attachment figure (the first listed feature) from distress (for example, manifest by anxiety, crying, and misery) in anticipation of separation from an attachment figure (another listed feature). ICD-10 criteria stipulated 'the criteria for generalized anxiety disorder of childhood are not met'; indicating that when they are present, the diagnosis of GAD should be preferred to separation anxiety disorder. It is also hard to distinguish between two other features relating to sleep disturbance, namely insomnia marked by persistent reluctance or refusal to go to sleep without being near an attachment figure, from the presence of repeated nightmares involving themes of separation.

Within ICD-11 criteria [5], the central psychopathological feature is the marked and excessive fear or anxiety about the separation of the individual from specific attachment figures, i.e., figures with whom they have a deep emotional bond: though clinical features vary according to developmental level. In children and adolescents, fear or anxiety concerns relate mainly to separation from caregivers, parents and/or other family members. These manifestations are judged to exceed what is considered a normal reaction at that developmental stage. In adults, symptoms mainly concern children and/or a romantic partner. However, they can be concerned with other close relationships (including parents or siblings, or even pets), with fears that the attachment figure may be exposed to harmful events, a reluctance or refusal to go to school or work due to these fears, and excessive distress when the subject is separated from the attachment figure. Patients' sleep function may be disrupted by recurrent nightmares about separation, and they may be reluctant or refuse to sleep away from the attachment figure: symptoms must persist for at least several months and be severe enough to cause significant distress and/or significant impairment in major areas of functioning for diagnostic criteria to be met. Compared to ICD-10, the use of ICD-11 criteria results in greater accuracy in diagnosing separation anxiety disorder (and other conditions) [6].

2 Epidemiology of Separation Anxiety Disorder in Adults

Separation anxiety symptoms are not infrequent across the lifespan. For example, a prospective study involving adolescents and young adults (aged 14–24 years) found a 7.8% 'lifetime prevalence' of separation anxiety symptoms [7]. An investigation in first-semester college students found that 21% met or exceeded the symptom threshold on a checklist of separation anxiety symptoms [8]. Approximately 25% of women attending a hospital ante-natal clinic had supra-threshold levels of separation anxiety [9], and marked separation anxiety was also present in approximately 35% of primiparous women whose unsettled infants had been admitted to a parent-child residential unit [10]. Taken together, these three studies [8–10] suggest that separation anxiety symptoms may be prominent during periods of transition through life stages. Furthermore, separation anxiety was found in around 3.5% of elderly (60 years or older) primary care patients [11]. However, recognizing the *symptoms* of separation anxiety does not necessarily indicate the presence of separation anxiety *disorder*, as its diagnosis also rests on evaluating the degree of personal distress and level of impairment.

In the US National Co-morbidity Survey Replication (NCS-R) epidemiological study (n = 5692), the estimated lifetime prevalence of separation anxiety disorder was 6.6%: the prevalence being higher in females than males, this difference being especially marked in the sub-group in whom separation anxiety started in childhood [12]. Although 36.1% of cases with an onset of separation anxiety in childhood experienced symptoms that persisted into adult life, the majority (77.5%) of cases in adults had an onset during adulthood. Adult separation anxiety disorder impairs social and work functioning markedly: more than 40% have severe impairment in at least one life domain, most commonly in the domains of social and personal life: impairment being more marked in those with comorbidity, which was present in more than half the cases in the NCS-R study [12].

Data from the World Health Organization (WHO) World Mental Health Surveys involving 18 countries indicate that the lifetime prevalence of separation anxiety disorder in the general population (n = 38,993 adults) has an average of 4.8%, with a rather broad interquartile range of 1.4–6.4%: 43.1% of lifetime onsets occurred in adulthood [13]. Rates of psychiatric comorbidity were similar to those in previous epidemiological studies. Evaluation of potential predictors of lifetime separation anxiety disorder identified female gender, reported childhood adversities, and lifetime traumatic events. These predicted separation anxiety disorder onsets in differing countries and in childhood, adolescence, and adulthood. A recent meta-analysis indicates that 72.4% and 75% of patients had an onset of illness by 14 and 18 years, respectively [14]: but at present, the typical duration of untreated illness in adult patients with separation anxiety disorder is unknown.

3 Distinguishing Separation Anxiety Disorder and Panic Disorder

Panic disorder is important in the differential diagnosis of separation anxiety disorder [15]: this distinction can be more difficult in patients with panic disorder with comorbid agoraphobia, among whom a history of separation anxiety disorder in childhood and adulthood is particularly common [16]. The main difference between adult separation anxiety disorder and panic disorder with agoraphobia is that in the former condition, the primary fear concerns potential separation from others (i.e., the concern is 'allocentric'), whereas the in the latter there is a persistent fear of having panic attacks (i.e., the concern is 'autocentric'). In adult patients with separation anxiety disorder, anxiety 'attacks' (if present) emerge within the context of potential or actual separation [1]. The main clinical characteristics of agoraphobia include a disproportionate fear of public places (such as shops or restaurants), often perceiving such an environment as too open, crowded or dangerous, resulting in psychological distress - and sometimes panic. Differential diagnosis between the conditions is aided by identifying the different situations that trigger the fear response and the reason why the individual fears of being alone in these situations: an agoraphobic patient typically fears that help will not be available, whereas a patient with separation anxiety disorder fears something bad might happen to a loved one, or that harm might happen whilst separated from a loved one. In children and adolescents, the main differentiating clinical feature is that in separation anxiety disorder, the concern relates to the potential loss of access to safe persons. In contrast, in panic disorder and agoraphobia, safety concerns involve a broad array of situations and environmental contexts [17].

In children with separation anxiety disorder, the major attachment figures are usually parents, and frequent separation behaviours include crying, tantrums, and school refusal or selective mutism. Adults with separation anxiety typically fear that some harm will affect their attachment figures (usually a spouse or child), so strenuous efforts are made to remain in close contact, despite marked impracticalities [18]. Childhood separation anxiety can be the primary condition in a trajectory of psychological illness manifesting as separation anxiety or other forms of mental disorder in young adults [19]. Early separation anxiety symptoms and behaviours can act as a 'general vulnerability factor', increasing the risk for anxiety and mood disorders in later years [20].

It seems reasonable to suppose that separation anxiety in adults was previously often erroneously construed as a form of panic disorder with or without agoraphobia [21]. By contrast, for many individuals, a diagnosis of adult separation anxiety disorder may have been more appropriate, with anxiety attacks being linked to threats of separation, rather than occurring unexpectedly or in feared situations, as in panic disorder. Differential diagnosis between separation anxiety disorder and panic disorder is aided by establishing that the fear of having a panic attack does not drive separation anxiety, whereas it does in agoraphobia: patients with separation anxiety disorder may experience panic attacks, but these are triggered by separations from close attachment figures, rather than being experienced as untriggered [4, 5], but the primary fear is the fear of separation, rather than the fear of having a panic attack [1]. More simplistically, a patient with panic disorder fears that a panic attack might result in a catastrophic event such as a 'heart attack', death, or going crazy or disappearing (or fainting), whereas a patient with separation anxiety disorder fears that if they have a heart attack, it might result in a hospital admission which would take them away from being close to their loved ones. In addition, patients with panic disorder are typically preoccupied with their personal health and safety, whereas individuals with separation anxiety disorder are primarily concerned for the well-being of their attachment figures (or sometimes themselves, should personal illness result in unwanted separation from others). The distinction of separation anxiety from agoraphobia is potentially complicated to parse, as at first blush it can appear that patients with separation anxiety are reluctant to venture out of their home. Agoraphobic situations are defined as places and situations from which escape might be difficult or in which help might not be available to the affected person; agoraphobic patients define magically 'safe' and 'dangerous' places often in relation to their homes, or what they imagine are easy escape routes to their homes. In separation anxiety disorder, the prominent fear is that something untoward might happen to someone else (loved ones or other major attachment figures) or that should they experience an untoward event, they could not be reunited with them [1].

4 Distinguishing Separation Anxiety Disorder from Other Conditions

Differential diagnosis between separation anxiety disorder and GAD can also be complex, as worrying that something bad might happen to a loved one is a feature common to the two conditions. Approximately half of children and adolescents with separation anxiety disorder worry about harm befalling their parents when not with them [22], and many children with the diagnosis of separation anxiety disorder also have a diagnosis of comorbid GAD [23]. The distinction between the two disorders in adults can also be difficult, but largely rests on establishing that the fear and persistent worry of losing loved ones is just one of a wide range of worrisome themes in patients with GAD (in which other common themes include personal health, financial concerns, and interpersonal difficulties); whereas in separation anxiety disorder, the central and often only concern is the fear of and intermittent worry about losing a major attachment figure [1]. Patients with GAD worry about significant others even though they are securely present, whereas patients with separation anxiety disorder feel relieved and worry less in the presence of their attachment figures.

The distinction between separation anxiety disorder and 'dependent personality disorder' is sometimes challenging. Dependent personality disorder is exemplified by a persistent, pervasive, and indiscriminate tendency to rely excessively on other individuals, particularly when making decisions. By contrast, separation anxiety disorder is characterized by a limited array of concerns about the proximity and safety of major attachment figures [18]. Adults with separation anxiety disorder typically report no difficulty in caring for themselves. Frantic efforts to avoid real or imagined abandonment are a feature of 'borderline personality disorder' but distinguishing between the two conditions is facilitated by identifying the pervasive mood instability and uncertainty with regards to self and most relationships, which is so troublesome in borderline personality disorder, but which is not a typical feature of separation anxiety disorder [2]. However, given how underdiagnosed SAD is in clinical settings, it is likely that some carrying the diagnosis of borderline personality disorder suffer from underlying separation anxiety disorder. Finally, a concern about the presumed misbehaviour of romantically attached figures is a feature of morbid jealousy, and this potentially hazardous condition should be included within the differential diagnosis, particularly when the worries and concerns about attachment figures have acquired a persistently preoccupying, obsessive, and querulous quality: however, little is established about how the conditions can be distinguished accurately.

5 Comorbidity in Separation Anxiety Disorder

Reliable diagnosis is made more difficult by the extensive comorbidity of separation anxiety disorder with other conditions established through a series of studies. For example, separation anxiety symptoms of both childhood-onset and adult-onset are common in patients with bipolar disorder, particularly those with an early onset [24]. Early separation anxiety is also common among women with eating disorders [25]. Separation anxiety *symptoms* are also common in outpatients with 'complicated grief' [26], or patients with post-traumatic stress disorder (PTSD) [27]. Furthermore, separation anxiety *disorder* was diagnosed in 56% of outpatients with affective disorders and complicated grief [28]: and features of prolonged grief, depression, and separation anxiety disorder were found to correlate significantly among bereaved individuals [29].

Observational studies in patients with obsessive compulsive disorder (OCD) have found a point prevalence of separation anxiety disorder of 27.2% [30], and a lifetime prevalence of 17% [31]. The relationship between separation anxiety and 'obsessivity' (as a personality trait rather than the diagnosis of OCD) is intriguing: existing data derive from examination of the relationship with insecure attachment, which finds an association between obsessiveness and high scores on the fearful dimension style of attachment, characterized by high levels of anxiety and avoidance [32]. Some adult individuals with separation anxiety may exert excessive control over relationships with significant figures (a core feature of obsessive compulsive personality disorder), with reticence towards unplanned changes in routine movements and trips: but more research is needed to clarify the nature of relationships between obsessional traits and separation anxiety symptoms. High separation anxiety or the diagnosis of separation anxiety disorder have been found to be associated with the presence of certain comorbid personality disorders (Clusters B and C) among patients attending an anxiety clinic [33].

6 Potential Mechanisms Underlying Adult Separation Anxiety Disorder

The aetiology of separation anxiety disorder in adults has not been explored extensively. The role of environmental and genetic factors and the ways in which they may interact is unclear [34]. Peripheral-type benzodiazepine binding site receptors, which have a role in the biosynthesis of steroids during stress and anxiety states, may have a significantly lower density in the sub-group of panic disorder patients in which coexisting separation anxiety is prominent [35]. Separation anxiety disorder appears associated with hypersensitivity to inhaled carbon dioxide [36]. Childhood separation anxiety disorder, adult panic disorder, and hypersensitivity to 35% carbon dioxide challenge may all share a common latent intervening variable [37–39]. However, not all evidence accords with this hypothesis, as children with separation anxiety disorder did not react with panic or increased anxiety symptoms after hyperventilation challenge when compared to controls with panic or other anxiety disorders [40].

Peripheral levels of the hypothalamic neuropeptide oxytocin (known to be involved in mother–infant interactions, and possibly involved in establishing trust in others) are potential biological markers of the dynamics of social relationships [41]. Children with separation anxiety disorder have been found to have significantly lower salivary oxytocin levels compared to children with other anxiety-related conditions [42]. However, mutation analysis of the oxytocin gene reveals no consistent disturbance in patients with adult separation anxiety disorder, although single nucleotide and intron two molecular variants have been detected [43]. A GG genotype single nucleotide polymorphism within the oxytocin receptor gene is linked to high levels of separation anxiety in patients with major depression [44].

7 Conclusions

Separation anxiety is a basic fear in humans, is readily observable in children, although generally becoming less prominent with age and maturity, and is underdiagnosed in adults. Marked separation anxiety probably represents a psychopathological phenomenon, and diagnostic criteria for separation anxiety disorder have benefitted from being progressively tightened. Including separation anxiety disorder within the group of anxiety disorders diagnosable in adults in DSM-5 and ICD-11 should encourage further research into its possibly distinctive phenotypes; and could identify possible endophenotypes delineating it from frequently comorbid conditions such as panic disorder, agoraphobia, and social anxiety disorder. Studies of the sensitivity of separation anxiety symptoms to carbon dioxide challenge, and of the potential role of oxytocin in dysfunctional attachment may provide fruitful in helping separate this common and burdensome condition from apparently similar conditions.

7.1 Clinical Case Example

Being the youngest member of a large, hard-working and loving family, Anne* was never alone or had any time to feel bored or listless during early childhood. One by one, her older sisters left school at the earliest opportunity to work in local factories or shops, all seeing little value in further education. Their successive departures from the family home to marry and live elsewhere in the city caused Anne to periodically question her previous determination to 'get on in life' by staying on at College, aiming to enter University. But she resolved to continue her studies, hoping for a nursing degree and subsequent employment as a paediatric nurse in the local hospital. Unfortunately, she found herself needing to repeat her second academic year (when 18 years old), as infectious mononucleosis ('glandular fever') and subsequent prolonged fatigue had made it hard to attend college or concentrate on allocated homework.

Knowing that Anne wished to enter University, and being worried about the financial implications of this, her mother decided to return to paid employment outside the home for the first time since the birth of her oldest child. This proved most unsettling for Anne, who was still recovering from fatigue. She feared for the health and safety of her mother at the tobacco-processing plant and on her long journeys to and from work on a public transport bus. Anne also became worried that if her illness were to take a turn for the worse, she would not be able to receive the loving care and support of her mother, whilst she was at the factory. She began to implore her mother to give up her new job, often expressing these concerns; and sometimes became tearful, angry and overtly upset as her mother prepared to leave the house to catch the early morning bus.

Her mother arranged for Anne to see their general practitioner (GP), who had known the family for many years. By this time, two of Anne's sisters had experienced periods of depression and undergone antidepressant treatment, and another had become markedly underweight and was drinking excessive quantities of alcohol. The GP took note of Anne's prolonged fatigue, tearfulness, and anxiety symptoms, and being aware of the family history of depression, made a diagnosis of depression. He prescribed a selective serotonin reuptake inhibitor (paroxetine) and referred Anne for counselling.

Anne could not tolerate paroxetine: she felt increasingly 'nervy' and it was becoming harder to sleep at night; and she declined the offer of counselling at the GP surgery, as this would have meant being away from her parents in the early evening, which made her anxious. Her concerns about potential untoward events affecting her mother steadily worsened, and at times she blocked the door, attempting to prevent mother from leaving the house. Surreptitiously, she began to follow her mother to work on a later bus, and took to regularly standing outside the tobacco plant, often for hours, hoping to glimpse her mother on the factory floor. When she was discovered doing this, her mother was embarrassed and exasperated, and criticized Anne for being 'stupid'. Anne could not keep up with the College homework, so had to withdraw from the course, thereby forsaking her intended future career as a nurse.

At this time, the GP referred Anne to the local community mental health service. She was diagnosed with panic disorder and agoraphobia, a diagnosis difficult to justify given these symptoms, prescribed another selective serotonin reuptake inhibitor (fluoxetine), and an enthusiastic mental health nurse instructed her in the techniques of *in vivo* desensitization giving Anne 'homework' to undertake, based on a constructed hierarchy of feared situations. Anne felt more agitated on fluoxetine and stopped it after a few days. She was also perplexed about the verbal and written instructions to expose herself to environments where she felt frightened, thinking this recommendation rather missed the point: her main concern was not of feeling anxious outside the family home, but instead about what might terrible things could happen to her mother whilst she was travelling to and working in the factory. Anne also became increasingly worried that her fatigue and anxiety could worsen and that there would be no-one to look after her should this happen, whilst her mother and father undertook their long working days. She stopped attending outpatient appointments.

Quite unexpectedly, Anne fell in love, with the son of long-standing friends of her parents. She and her boyfriend were soon engaged and Anne left the family home, once she discovered she was pregnant. She found it curious that her previous concerns about her mother had disappeared so rapidly. Sadly, this relief was only short-lived, as she soon began to make demands on her fiancé, begging him to work from home rather than travel to his office. She feared he might be involved in an accident whilst driving, or be unable to return swiftly, should she develop any acute problems during her pregnancy. The couple discussed the strain that these concerns were placing on their relationship at what should have been an enjoyable period and agreed that Anne should be referred again to the community mental health team. Anne did not wish to burden the relationship with her fiancé, neither did she want her future child to grow up having to cope with a troubled and dependent mother.

Reorganization of local mental health services had led to an innovative system for assessing patients with anxiety and depression: now, all were interviewed jointly by a trainee psychiatrist and trainee clinical psychologist, followed by subsequent discussion within a wider multi-disciplinary team. The initial interview had queried the initial diagnosis of panic disorder with agoraphobia, and after the discussion it was felt that adult-onset adult separation anxiety disorder was more likely: this revised diagnosis was confirmed in a subsequent interview with an experienced consultant psychiatrist.

Anne decided to defer pharmacological treatment until after her daughter was born, also choosing not to breast-feed. As she had not tolerated treatment with either of two selective serotonin reuptake inhibitors, she was prescribed the tricyclic anti-depressant clomipramine, its dosage being increased steadily from 25 mg/day to 150 mg/day. Initial drowsiness resolved quickly and Anne had no sense of increased nervousness, although she needed to be careful with her diet as she developed a liking for sweet foods and wanted to return to her pre-pregnant weight. She attended group therapy sessions focused on confidence-building and assertiveness-training and then undertook individual cognitive behaviour therapy which allowed her to examine the relationships between her thoughts, feelings and actions. Her husband gradually assumed greater responsibilities at work, and travels regularly around the country conducting site visits. Anne subsequently enrolled in a book-keeping course, obtained the professional qualifications, and now works as a freelance with a particular interest in small companies which support young mothers.

* The name and some autobiographic details have been changed, to prevent identification.

Acknowledgement DSB and VM are members of the Anxiety Disorders Research Network (ADRN), a component of the European College of Neuropsychopharmacology Network Initiative (ECNP-NI).

References

1. Bagels SM, Knappe S, Clark LA. Adult separation anxiety disorder in DSM-5. Clin Psychol Rev. 2013;33:663–74.
2. Manicavasagar V, Marnane C, Pini S, Abelli M, Rees S, Eapen V, Silove D. Adult separation anxiety disorder: a disorder comes of age. Curr Psychiatr Rep. 2010;12:290–7.
3. American Psychiatric Association. Diagnostic and Statistical Manual of Mental Disorders (DSM-5). Washington, DC: American Psychiatric Pub; 2013.
4. World Health Organization. The ICD-10 classification of mental and behavioural disorders. Diagnostic criteria for research. Geneva: World Health Organization; 1993.
5. World Health Organization. ICD-11: International classification of diseases (11th revision). Geneva: World Health Organization; 2019.
6. Rebello TJ, et al. Anxiety and fear-related disorders in the ICD-11: results from a global case-controlled field study. Arch Med Res. 2019;50:490–501.
7. Brückl TM, Wittchen H-U, Höfler M, Pfister H, Scheider S, Lieb R. Childhood separation anxiety and the risk of subsequent psychopathology: results from a community study. Psychother Psychosom. 2007;76:47–56.
8. Seligman LD, Wuyek LA. Correlates of separation anxiety symptoms among first-semester college students: an exploratory study. J Psychol. 2007;141:135–45.
9. Eapen V, Silove DM, Johnston D, Apler A, Rees S. Adult separation anxiety in pregnancy: how common is it? Int J Women's Health. 2012;4:251–6.
10. Kohlhoff J, Barnett B, Eapen V. Adult separation anxiety and unsettled infant behaviour: associations with adverse parenting during childhood and insecure adult attachment. Compr Psychiatry. 2015;61:1–9.
11. Wijeratne C, Manicavasagar V. Separation anxiety in the elderly. J Anxiety Disord. 2003;17:695–702.
12. Shear K, Jin R, Ruscio AM, Walters EE, Kessler RC. Prevalence and correlates of estimated DSM- IV child and adult separation anxiety disorder in the national comorbidity survey replication. Am J Psychiatr. 2006;163:1074–83.
13. Silove D, Alonso J, Bromet E, Gruber M, Sampson N, Scott K, Andrade L, Benjet C, Caldas de Almeida JM, De Girolamo G, de Jonge P, Demyttenaere K, Fiestas F, Florescu S, Gureje O, He Y, Karam E, Lepine JP, Murphy S, Villa-Posada J, Zarkov Z, Kessler RC. Pediatric-onset and adult-onset separation anxiety disorder across countries in the World Mental Health Survey. Am J Psychiatry. 2015;172:647–56.
14. Solmi M, Radua J, Olivola M, Croce E, Soardo L, de Pablo S, et al. Age at onset of mental disorders worldwide: large-scale meta-analysis of 192 epidemiological studies. Mol Psychiatry. 2022;27:281–95.
15. Silove DM, Marnane C. Overlap of symptom domains of separation anxiety disorder in adulthood with panic disorder-agoraphobia. J Anxiety Disord. 2013;27:92–7.
16. Dogan B, Kocabas O, Sevincok D, et al. Separation anxiety disorder in panic disorder patients with and without agoraphobia. Psychiatry. 2021;84:66–80.
17. Eisen AR, Toffey KL. Separation anxiety disorder. In: Olatunji BO, editor. The Cambridge handbook of anxiety and related disorders. Cambridge: Cambridge University Press; 2019.
18. Pini S, Abelli M, Shear KM, Cardini A, Lari L, Gesi C, Muti M, Calugi S, Galderisi S, Troisi A, Bertolino A, Cassano GB. Frequency and clinical correlates of adult separation anxiety in a sample of 508 outpatients with mood and anxiety disorders. Acta Psychiatr Scand. 2010;122:40–6.

19. Lewinsohn PM, Holm-Denoma JM, Small JW, Seeley JR, Joiner TE. Separation anxiety disorder in childhood as a risk factor for future mental illness. J Am Acad Child Adolesc Psychiatry. 2008;47:548–55.
20. Kossowsky J, Pfaltz MC, Schneider S, Taeymans J, Locher C, Gaab J. The separation anxiety hypothesis of panic disorder revisited: a meta-analysis. Am J Psychiatry. 2013;170:768–81.
21. Silove DM, Rees S. Separation anxiety disorder across the lifespan: DSM-5 lifts age restriction on diagnosis. Asian J Psychiatr. 2014;11:98–101.
22. Masi G, Mucci M, Favilla L, Romano R, Poli P. Symptomatology and comorbidity of generalized anxiety disorder in children and adolescents. Compr Psychiatry. 1999;3:210–5.
23. Verduin TL, Kendall P. Differential occurrence of comorbidity within childhood anxiety disorders. J Clin Child Adolesc Psychiatry. 2003;2:290–5.
24. Pini S, Abelli M, Mauri M, Muti M, Iazzetta P, Banti S, Cassano GB. Clinical correlates and significance of separation anxiety in patients with bipolar disorder. Bipolar Disord. 2005;7:370–6.
25. Troisi A, Massaroni P, Cuzzolaro M. Early separation anxiety and adult attachment style in women with eating disorders. Br J Clin Psychol. 2005;44:89–97.
26. Dell'Osso L, Carmassi C, Corsi M, Pergentini I, Socci C, Maremmani AGI, Perugi G. Adult separation anxiety in patients with complicated grief versus healthy control subjects: relationships with lifetime depressive and hypomanic symptoms. Ann Gen Psychiatry. 2011;10:29.
27. Dell'Osso L, Carmassi C, Musetti L, Socci C, Shear MK, Conversano C, Maremmani I, Perugi G. Lifetime mood symptoms and adult separation anxiety in patients with complicated grief and/or post-traumatic stress disorder: a preliminary report. Psychiatry Res. 2012;198:436–40.
28. Pini S, Gesi C, Abelli M, Muti M, Lari L, Cardini A, Manicavasagar V, Mauri M, Cassano GB, Shear KM. The relationship between adult separation anxiety disorder and complicated grief in a cohort of 454 outpatients with mood and anxiety disorders. J Affect Disord. 2012;143:64–8.
29. Boelen PA. Symptoms of prolonged grief, depression, and adult separation anxiety: distinctiveness and correlates. Psychiatry Res. 2013;207:68–72.
30. Franz AP, Rateke L, Hartmann T, McLaughlin N, Torres AR, do Rosario MC, Filho ECM, Ferrão YA. Separation anxiety disorder in adult patients with obsessive-compulsive disorder: prevalence and clinical correlates. Eur Psychiatry. 2015;30:145–51.
31. Mroczkowski MM, Goes FS, Riddle MA, Grados MA, Bievenu OJ, Greenberg BD, Fyer AJ, et al. Separation anxiety disorder in OCD. Depress Anxiety. 2011;28:256–62.
32. Wiltgen A, Adler H, Smith R, Rufino K, Frazier C, Shepard C, Booker K, Simmons D, Richardson L, Allen JG, Fowler JC. Attachment insecurity and obsessive-compulsive personality disorder among inpatients with serious mental illness. J Affect Disord. 2015;174:411–5.
33. Silove DM, Marnane CL, Wagner R, Manicavasagar VL. Associations of personality disorder with early separation anxiety in patients with adult separation anxiety disorder. J Pers Disord. 2010;25:128–33.
34. Scaini S, Ogliari A, Eley TC, Zavos HMS, Battaglia M. Genetic and environment contributions to separation anxiety: a meta-analytic approach to twin data. Depress Anxiety. 2012;29:754–61.
35. Pini S, Martini C, Abelli M, Muti M, Gesi C, Montali M, Chelli B, Lucacchini A, Cassano GB. Peripheral-type benzodiazepine receptor binding sites in platelets of patients with panic disorder associated to separation anxiety symptoms. Psychopharmacology. 2005;181:407–11.
36. Atli O, Bayin M, Alkin T. Hypersensitivity to 35% carbon dioxide in patients with adult separation anxiety disorder. J Affect Disord. 2012;141:315–23.
37. Roberson-Nay R, Klein DF, Klein RG, Mannuzza S, Moulton JL, Guardino M, Pine DS. Carbon dioxide hypersensitivity in separation-anxious offspring of parents with panic disorder. Biol Psychiatry. 2010;67:1171–7.
38. Roberson-Nay R, Eaves LJ, Hettema JM, Kendler KS, Silberg JL. Childhood separation anxiety disorder and adult onset panic attacks share a common genetic diathesis. Depress Anxiety. 2012;29:320–7.
39. Battaglia M, Pesenti-Gritti P, Medland SE, Ogliari A, Tambs K, Spatola CAM. A genetically informed study of the association between childhood separation anxiety, sensitivity to CO_2, panic disorder, and the effect of childhood parental loss. Arch Gen Psychiatry. 2009;66:64–71.

40. Kossowsky J, Wilhem FH, Schneider S. Response to voluntary hyperventilation in children with separation anxiety disorder: implications for the link to panic disorder. J Anxiety Disord. 2013;27:627–34.
41. Crockford C, Deschner T, Ziegler TE, Witting RM. Endogenous peripheral oxytocin measures can give insight into the dynamics of social relationships: a review. Front Behav Neurosci. 2014;8:68.
42. Lebowitz ER, Leckmand JF, Feldman R, Zagoory-Sharon O, McDonald N, Silverman WK. Salivary oxytocin in clinically anxious youth: associations with separation anxiety and family accommodation. Psychoneuroendocrinology. 2016;65:35–43.
43. Costa B, Pini S, Martini C, Abelli M, Gabelloni P, Ciampi O, Muti M, Gesi C, Lari L, Cardini A, Mucci A, Bucci P, Lucacchini A, Cassano GB. Mutation analysis of oxytocin gene in individuals with adult separation anxiety. Psychiatry Res. 2009;168:87–93.
44. Costa B, Pini S, Gabelloni P, Abelli M, Lari L, Cardini A, Muti M, Gesi C, Landi S, Galderisi S, Mucci A, Lucacchini A, Cassano GB, Martini C. Oxytocin receptor polymorphisms and adult attachment style in patients with depression. Psychoneuroendocrinology. 2009;10:1506–14.

Clinical Case Descriptions and Discussion

Stefano Pini and Barbara Milrod

1 Separation Anxiety Leading to Panic Disorder

Lara was a 28-year-old unmarried bisexual woman who suddenly, apparently out of the blue, developed crippling panic attacks in which she felt herself disappearing or "flying into space." During panic episodes, which initially felt as though they came "out of the blue," it took her hours to calm down, and she felt unable to be alone for even one minute. She also suddenly developed severe agoraphobia such that she required a friend or family member to take her every single place she needed to go (a phobic companion), including to her therapist, or to work. While she had always been unable to stay alone at night since earliest childhood because of severe separation anxiety, Lara's inability to be alone became much worse when panic attacks started, several years before presenting for treatment.

Panic started one afternoon when she was sitting in her car, waiting for a friend to come downstairs to start off on the drive in which she was moving from her old apartment into her new apartment. Lara had the sudden onset of severe panic accompanied by a sense of unreality, depersonalization, and doom. She felt disconnected from her body. The symptoms lasted for hours, and her friend, who had been helping her to pack, needed to drive her to the new apartment and stay with her. At the time, Lara was moving from an apartment she had shared with her ex-girlfriend, Melissa, who had been abusive to her, into another apartment with her girlfriend, Emily. Before her severe panic episode, Lara was unsure whether she wanted her

S. Pini
Department of Clinical and Experimental Medicine, University of Pisa, Pisa, Italy
e-mail: stefano.pini@unipi.it

B. Milrod (✉)
Psychiatry and Behavioral Science (PRIME), Albert Einstein College of Medicine, New York, NY, USA
e-mail: bmilrod@montefiore.org

S. Pini, B. Milrod (eds.), *Separation Anxiety in Adulthood*,
https://doi.org/10.1007/978-3-031-37446-3_9

relationship with Emily to be romantic. She reported that it was difficult for her to judge what she wanted from relationships, and her panic attacks and terror of being alone and feeling "lost" clouded the picture. After the experience of the disorganizing panic attack in her car, Lara had trouble driving while alone "because I feel I could lose myself," making commuting from her home to her graduate school or to her job nearly impossible. Suddenly, paradoxically, while she thought she was on the cusp of breaking free from a controlling, abusive relationship, Lara found herself unable to function alone.

While panic attacks and agoraphobia were relatively new to her, Lara suffered from severe separation anxiety throughout most of her life. She had been (and remained to a great extent) highly separation anxious from her mother and remembered being "glued" to her throughout her childhood and until she had finally managed to enroll in college two towns away from where mother was living. In a famous story from early childhood, Lara's mother had left Lara with her grandmother for a few days to visit her sister in San Francisco, and Lara had become so upset and ill, vomiting, and unable to sleep for fear her mother would die, that mother was obliged to return home and bring Lara with her for the remainder of the trip. Lara slept in bed with mother until she was 6 years old.

Her parents had a tumultuous relationship with a lot of loud fighting that ended in divorce when Lara was 6. Lara reported that she never felt "safe" with her father, even though she loved him. Mother was highly anxious herself, and was particularly preoccupied with Lara's health, and Lara remembered mother waking her to "check" on her multiple times each night to make sure she "was still breathing." Lara's younger sister was born when Lara was 5 years old, and Lara felt responsible for taking good care of her sister from an early age. Lara felt her mother was unstable and dangerous, at risk herself because of her alcohol use and string of abusive boyfriends, and she worried that mother would be unable to help her sister or herself if they became ill. Lara recalled having the conviction that if she did not watch Nancy, something bad might happen to her. "My mother was too much of a wreck to take care of her." Lara and Nancy shared a bed from the time Nancy was 16 months old; they moved out of mother's bed at the time of her parents' divorce, when mother almost immediately brought in a new live-in boyfriend. "At least I knew Nancy would be OK if I was physically right next to her," Lara said.

Lara recalled abortive sleep-over dates throughout elementary and middle school in which she suddenly became terrified that her mother would not take good enough care of her sister. She would wind up terrified, demanding to be taken home before bedtime. Thus, well before panic onset, and years before her sense of inability to go anywhere alone, Lara's relationships with those closest to her were characterized by a chronic sense of danger and terror of separations from mother or sister, with the ominous sense that something terrible, potentially even life threatening, could happen to her or her sister if they were not all together all the time. Paradoxically, during childhood, Lara had felt like "the only competent one" in her family, yet since panic, she suddenly felt unable to even care for herself.

Lara's premorbid separation anxiety was extreme: she had always been frightened to spend a single night in a bed alone. She went from sleeping with mother to sleeping with her sister every night. When she left for a nearby college, she instantly began sleeping in a bed with her roommate. This terror of sleeping alone in a bed at night led to extreme complications and tumultuousness in her romantic life, with Lara seeming to bounce from partner to partner (or to having multiple partners at once) in an effort to have a companion in bed.

1.1 Discussion

The backdrop of Lara's terrifying/dangerous attachment relationships, in which all relationships came to be imbued with a sense of danger, originating both with mother's anxious terror about her health, as well as the fraught and explosive relationship between her parents, paved the way for Lara to become involved in an abusive, controlling relationship with her ex-girlfriend. Despite the abusive qualities of this relationship (the ex-girlfriend would not "permit" Lara to see her family without her also being present, for example), Lara had come to depend on her for a sense of personal safety. This underlying terror of separation and feeling of personal instability also made breaking up with the ex-girlfriend, a decision she had considered seriously over time, feel as though she were losing control of herself. Lara's highly separation anxious backdrop played a key role in the explosive emergence of her panic disorder and agoraphobia, and required specific psychotherapeutic focus in order for her to achieve remission. This patient met SCID-II [1] criteria for comorbid borderline personality disorder at the time of her presentation, (the patient presented with primary DSM panic disorder with severe agoraphobia). This patient's fluctuating and chaotic relationship patterns were better understandable, however, as arising from her profound separation anxiety disorder and the burden placed on all of her close relationships because she could not sleep alone. This case is illustrative in the way underlying, profound separation anxiety leads to panic disorder, severe agoraphobia, and even comorbid borderline personality disorder.

2 Separation Anxiety Underlying Childhood Depression

Alex is a 22-year-old single man living in Livorno. He is the son of a judge. His parents were separated for 6 years but had reunited 2 years ago, at a time that coincided with Alex's developing major depression. The patient's premorbid personality is vividly recalled by him as having a tendency to melancholy and isolation when away from home, but a sense of well-being when at home with his parents. He recalls discomfort, anxiety, and sadness when away from both parents as a child. He never managed to have close friends, and reported few, fairly distant social relationships. At about 20 years of age, Alex developed symptoms characterized by a decline in mood, anhedonia, classic diurnal variation, asthenia, apathy, social withdrawal, he spent all of his time in bed, increased appetite, and hypersomnia. Just before the patient became depressed, his father, who had separated from his wife 6 years earlier because he had fallen in love with another woman, returned to his wife and the family home. This intense response to his father's return to his mother was surprising, because Alex's relationship with his father had remained, at least on the surface, very good throughout his parents' separation. The two had continued to see each other and spent a lot of time together, especially during the summer holidays, although Alex had never accepted his father's new girlfriend and had steadfastly refused to establish any relationship with her.

When he became depressed, Alex was in London for a few months for a work experience planned for about a year. Both parents, especially his mother, encouraged him to go to London. From ages 16 to about 19, he struggled with a substance abuse disorder which the patient felt was not interfering with his life. The cannabinoid abuse was continuous over time, while those of ecstasy, cocaine, and LSD were limited to a few sporadic episodes.

Upon his return to Italy, the patient had a slow and gradual worsening of depression, manifested by mild withdrawal to social isolation, a marked sensitivity to separations from his mother, severe anxiety, and reduced frustration tolerance. Despite these symptoms, he was able to start and maintain a relationship with a girl, Micaela.

For 2 years, the patient was followed by a specialist and took antidepressant medication and significantly improved. However, when Micaela broke up with him, he became depressed again and ruminated about the breakup. Since then, he has been followed in the clinic, receiving both pharmacotherapy and psychotherapy, which has helped him to be able to enroll in university and function better.

In therapy, Alex always maintained that he believed in order to avoid hurting him, his father had initially tried to hide his new romantic relationship from him. Alex had interpreted this behavior as a lack of respect toward him. After 6 years apart, his father reunited with his wife and returned to the original family nucleus.

At his first presentation, Alex was depressed and obsessively ruminating about his recent breakup. Micaela had left him, and although he claimed never to have been in love with her, he could not tolerate that she abandoned him. He reported feelings of loneliness and sadness, and unbearable feelings of rejection. He said he now lived with a continuous sense of abandonment and intense separation anxiety from Micaela.

Alex also suffered from mood swings: moments of irritability and dysphoric mood with worsening symptoms toward the evening. The patient's past and current interpersonal relationships and their relationship to the present depressive symptoms were considered. In particular, it relatively rapidly emerged that Alex's current depressive picture was emotionally linked to an unstated, barely acknowledged interpersonal conflict with his father, aggravated by the pain he was experiencing in mourning his relationship with Micaela. Another element that may have contributed to his developing depression was the transition he felt in his role from his exclusive relationship with his mother to the greater distance and separation from her of his new role as an adult son in his home with his father's return.

With disgust, Alex described his father as anxious, weak, and insecure, almost dependent on his wife. His rage at his father came to the fore: Alex focused on how father behaved as a hypocrite and a liar when he left his mother, he had never even dared to tell him the truth. In addition, the patient did not appreciate his return to the family. He considered this gesture to have arisen from opportunism and his father's psychological incompetence and dependence on his mother. It might also have felt to Alex that he had been functioning as the man of the house when his father left, and he felt usurped, experiencing his father's return as another kind of loss. In either case, when he became depressed, Alex felt an extreme need for proximity to his mother, although he initially had difficulties recognizing or acknowledging this.

Alex described his mother as a strong and energetic woman, autonomous and independent, endowed with excellent ability in social relationships, and toward whom the patient has deep esteem and has always confided and shared all his life experiences. The patient reported having a better relationship with his mother than his father. His mother had always proved to be understanding and available to help him in moments of difficulty when his depressive symptoms reappeared, father tended to cut out.

Alex's father, who organized Alex's psychiatric care and physically accompanied him to his first psychiatric visit, was hoping for a better relationship with his son. Father was physically demonstrative with Alex, with kisses, caresses, and pats on the shoulder, behaviors that Alex refused to reciprocate and found enraging, saying he was no longer a child.

Initially, Alex did not recognize that his depression had always emerged in relationship to core separations: (first, at about 14 years of age when his parents separated and his father left home, at about 20 when his parents reunited and he moved away from home to London, and then, most recently, during the tumultuous breakup with Micaela when she left him, which became even more acute when he struggled desperately to prolong the relationship).

Alex would not discuss his relationship with Micaela with his psychiatrist. If asked direct questions, he replied concisely and dryly, claiming that he was never in love with her but had tolerated abandonment badly. However, Alex did say that he did not understand the reason for the breakup, and assumed that Micaela was tired of having a relationship with a depressed, apathetic person without initiative who is plagued by emotional outbursts, even though she had been close to him for a long time and had helped him through his past depression. He said he thought that the object of his brooding was not the loss of Micaela *per se*, but the affront that she gave him by leaving him. After the breakup, despite his depression, Alex claimed to have complete disinterest in her.

2.1 Discussion

The case of Alex illustrates the way in which underlying separation anxiety sets up a person for longstanding global difficulty in forming relationships outside of the home. Then later, separations and disruptions in close attachment relationships through the course of life serve as aggravating triggers for more profound depression and mood disturbances. For Alex, who evidently had underlying separation anxiety before he experienced key separations in his relationships, the three important separations that triggered his depressions were when his father left his mother (and him), which felt like a betrayal and abandonment to Alex, when he left home and his mother to live in London, and when Micaela left him. This case illustrates how Alex views his own separation anxiety as an embarrassing and disgraceful weakness, making it more difficult to approach and focus on in treatment. He denigrates his attachment figures (father, Michaela) other than his mother, who he views as "strong." He is particularly disgusted with his father for his return to his mother, and describes him as "shamefully" dependent on his mother. He repudiates him for this, brushing off his "childish" kisses, with the feeling of revulsion that he might be demonstrating similar separation/attachment conflicts. There is the sense that such feelings and struggles are perceived as unmanly. He is furious and denigrating toward those who have left him (father, Micaela). Evidently, being able to tolerate the idea that he suffers from separation anxiety himself will require some work in psychotherapy in order for him to tolerate any of his feelings.

3 Separation Anxiety Disorder in a Patient with Suicidal Behavior Disorder Admitted to an Intensive Care Unit

Marianna is a 40-year-old divorced woman with two small children who attempted suicide, ingesting hydrochloric acid and medications (trazodone and benzodiazepines). She was psychiatrically evaluated after she was admitted to the University Hospital Intensive Care Unit (ICU). Physically, she had severe oral and esophageal damage, and several hematologic abnormalities due to the toxic effects of the ingestion. She had attempted suicide impulsively, swallowing the hydrochloric acid and drugs in the bathroom while her two daughters, aged 6 and 8, watched television in the living room. Marianna was found vomiting in the bedroom by her older daughter an hour later. Her daughter called EMS. She was admitted to a local first aid center and transferred to the ICU, awaiting surgical intervention for her esophageal perforations. During her ICU stay, she was evaluated by the liaison psychiatrists, who followed her during the hospitalization. On her first mental status examination at admission, she was somewhat confused, disoriented to place and time, with difficulties in attention. She was not able to cooperate during the interview.

The suicide attempt occurred after a romantic breakup one month earlier, as reported by the patient and her mother. After the breakup, she spent about a month with increased energy levels (subjective and as observed by her mother), a decreased need for sleep, ruminations about the breakup, seeking proximity to her ex-boyfriend, and mood instability. During this period, she also neglected the hygiene and nutrition of her two daughters. The patient did not have a clear-cut diagnosed mood disorder or frank psychiatric disorder in the past, although she is reported to have taken psychotropic medication since age 30. Marianna had attempted suicide in the past, ingesting drugs (benzodiazepines), five years earlier, after her divorce from her husband, another significant loss/separation event.

According to her mother, Marianna had never had any symptoms of separation anxiety in childhood. She appeared to develop separation anxiety symptoms from her mother after she got married and left home at age 30. A clear-cut psychiatric diagnosis did not emerge during the initial evaluation. However, she described periods of mood instability since a young age, with occasional episodes of intense anxiety and frequent use of benzodiazepines. On further follow-up evaluation, the nature of some previously untreated mood episodes emerged more clearly with additional information provided by the mother. The most plausible long-term baseline mood disorder backdrop for this patient was cyclothymia.

For Marianna, a solid temporal correlation rapidly emerged between important separation triggers and events and more severe bipolar spectrum episodes, which, both in the case of her divorce from her husband and her current breakup, reached the level of mixed bipolar/manic episodes.

3.1 Discussion

In both Marianna's and Alex's cases described above, underlying separation sensitivity, and in Alex's case, underlying separation anxiety disorder since childhood, serves as a backdrop for later presentation with frank DSM major mood disorders. Triggers, predictably, revolve around interpersonal loss events and separations from core attachment objects. While the major mood episodes require appropriate pharmacological and psychotherapeutic treatment, patients remain vulnerable to recurrences until the organizing separation anxiety that underlies their emotional life can be articulated, understood, and thoroughly addressed in therapy.

Reference

1. First MB, Spitzer RL, Gibbon M et al. Structured clinical interview for DSM-IV Axis II personality disorders (Version 2.0) Biometrics Research Department, NY State Psychiatric Institute, 722 West 168th Street New York, N.Y. 10032.

Conclusions

Stefano Pini and Barbara Milrod

For much of its history, separation anxiety has been a relatively neglected domain in psychiatry. Lifting the age restriction (<18 years in DSM-IV) on the diagnosis of SAD reflects the increasing evidence that disorder onset is not limited to childhood or adolescence, but often first manifests during adulthood.

Epidemiological data revealed a high lifetime prevalence of childhood-onset SAD (CSAD) of about 4%, but a higher lifetime prevalence of 6.1% for adult-onset SAD (ASAD), with 36.1% of childhood-onset cases persisting into adulthood and as many as 77.5% of adult cases reporting first onset after the age of 18. Childhood prevalence rates are higher in girls than boys, although sex differences are less pronounced in adulthood. However, men are more likely to report disorder onset during adulthood. SAD appears to be highly comorbid with and antecedent to other mental disorders, including anxiety disorders, depression and bipolar disorder, stress-related disorders, and personality disorders. Including SAD in the group of anxiety disorders and thereby lifting the age limit in the DSM-5 has renewed research efforts into its epidemiology and etiology. Surely, separation anxiety has been shown to complicate the course and severity of these comorbid disorders. This may in part pertain to the elucidation of neurobiological mechanisms, which on the one hand, may constitute stable risk factors of SAD across age groups, and, on the other hand, act as neutral, adaptive or maladaptive markers depending on different time windows of age.

S. Pini (✉)
Department of Clinical and Experimental Medicine, University of Pisa, Pisa, Italy
e-mail: stefano.pini@unipi.it

B. Milrod
Psychiatry and Behavioral Science (PRIME), Albert Einstein College of Medicine, New York, NY, USA
e-mail: bmilrod@montefiore.org

S. Pini, B. Milrod (eds.), *Separation Anxiety in Adulthood*,
https://doi.org/10.1007/978-3-031-37446-3_10

We approached this book with the clinician in mind. Throughout, we have emphasized the clinical implications of current research while also seeking to provide critical reviews to stimulate further research developments.

This book reflects the crossroads at which we currently stand: the very provisional status of our theoretical map, our frustration with achieving good outcomes clinically with people afflicted by separation anxiety disorder into adulthood, and some basic unresolved questions.

Is a reliable and valid taxonomy of anxiety disorders possible that considers the role and impact of separation anxiety? Can contemporary heuristic approaches to axis I mental health problems, as many still call them, be adapted for separation anxiety as a clinically meaningful entity (as has happened with psychotherapies), or do we need new approaches?

How can psychiatrists and psychologists reconcile their biopsychosocial formulations with the ramifications of separation anxiety disorder as a diagnosis that, originating from the realm of attachment theory, is now considered a condition with equal relevance as other mental disorders? The ramifications and complexity of attachment relationships and their implications for emotional development have been difficult to assimilate into the more phenomenologically-driven realm of general psychiatric nosology. However, attachment remains crucial to mental health, severity of psychopathology, and what goes into our understanding of which patients have more promising vs. less promising prognoses.

How much of the clinical and theoretical consensus that has crept into classification systems and contemporary practice will stand the test of systematic research in this area over the next few decades? Incorporating attachment and development into the realm of psychiatric nosology carries some hope with it of greater understanding. Sadly, because of psychoanalysis' long history of eschewing systematic research and maintaining a literature separate from mainstream mental health literature [1, 2], theoretical constructs such as classical psychoanalytically-derived object relations theory did not stimulate systematic empirical research. This represents a lost opportunity. The problem is not that theories are necessarily wrong but rather that they remain untested. Although elements of the separation anxiety syndrome are captured by parts some of these theories [3, 4], they do not incorporate essential developments elucidating psychopathological trajectories that pertain to separation anxiety as is currently understood.

For these reasons, it was decided to organize the volume around key topics rather than to allow contemporary models to impose a structure that is justified by the evidence available, which in many domains is inadequate to make definitive statements. The intention is to provide a systematic account of empirical knowledge that is as little concentrated as possible by unsubstantiated assumptions of traditional models and theories while at the same time recognizing their importance. The focus of this book is on empirical knowledge and the implications it has for both theory and practice in working with patients who clinically suffer from separation anxiety.

References

1. Busch FN, Milrod B. The ongoing struggle for psychoanalytic research: some steps forward. Psychoanal Psychother. 2010;24:306–14.
2. Milrod B, Busch F. Problems facing researchers in psychoanalysis. Psychoanal Inq. 2003;23:211–7.
3. Bowlby J. Separation anxiety: a critical review of the literature. J Child Psychol Psychiatry. 1960;1:231–26.
4. Mahler MS. On human symbiosis and the vicissitudes of individuation, Infantile psychosis, vol. 1. New York: International Universities Press; 1968. 1969

MIX
Papier aus verantwortungsvollen Quellen
Paper from responsible sources
FSC® C105338

If you have any concerns about our products,
you can contact us on
ProductSafety@springernature.com

In case Publisher is established outside the EU,
the EU authorized representative is:
Springer Nature Customer Service Center GmbH
Europaplatz 3, 69115 Heidelberg, Germany

Printed by Libri Plureos GmbH
in Hamburg, Germany